# Homoeopathic Science & Modern Medicine

## THE PHYSICS OF HEALING WITH MICRODOSES

# Harris L. Coulter, Ph.D.

**With an addendum on case-taking by James Tyler Kent, M.D.**

NORTH ATLANTIC BOOKS, BERKELEY, CALIFORNIA

Acknowledgements

The preface "Homoeopathy Revisited" was reprinted with permission from *Centerscope*, a publication of Boston University Medical Center (September-October, 1970).

The text of this book was originally published as "Homoeopathy and Modern Medical Science," *Journal of the American Institute of Homeopathy* (three parts) June, September, December, 1980 (73, 2–4).

The preface and the text were both rewritten specially for this publication.

Homoeopathic Science and Modern Medicine
by Harris L. Coulter, Ph.D.

ISBN 0-913028-84-3 (paperback)
ISBN 0-913028-86-X (limited edition hardcover)

*Publishers' Addresses:*

North Atlantic Books
2800 Woolsey Street
Berkeley, California 94705

Homoeopathic Educational Services
2124 Kittredge Street
Berkeley, California 94704

Cover design by Paula Morrison

**Homoeopathic Science and Modern Medicine** is sponsored by the Society for the Study of Native Arts and Sciences, a nonprofit educational corporation whose goals are to develop an ecological and crosscultural perspective linking various scientific, social, and artistic fields; to nurture a holistic view of arts, sciences, humanities, and healing; and to publish and distribute literature on the relationship of mind, body, and nature.

# Contents

# *Preface*
# Homoeopathy Revisited

The homoeopathic movement is one of the most intriguing phenomena in the history of medicine. Since the doctrine was announced in the early 1800's by its originator, Samuel Hahnemann (1755-1843), there has at all times been a group of physicians who, although trained in the accepted approach to medicine and healing, have nonetheless preferred the homoeopathic alternative. This alternative consists of a series of therapeutic assumptions which are entirely opposed to the basic tenets of orthodox medicine (by "orthodox" medicine we mean the "scientific" medical tradition of the nineteenth and twentieth centuries—also known as allopathy). For 180 years the practitioners of homoeopathy have refused to be integrated into the orthodox tradition and have led an autonomous existence somewhere on the fringe of medical thought and practice.

The existence of this competing group has always been a source of peculiar discomfiture to medical orthodoxy. Regular physicians could regard with equanimity the various attacks of uneducated practitioners, but the homoeopaths from the very beginning have been at least as well educated as the regular physicians themselves. Most are graduates of the orthodox schools and know orthodox medicine from the inside.

1

At the same time they have been strongly critical of the orthodox procedures.

Because medical orthodoxy since Hahnemann's day (and before) has regarded its own doctrines as "scientific," and hence not susceptible of fundamental theoretical reconstruction, these practitioners could never grant recognition to a doctrine which attacked the very foundations of their system of practice. They could not take a dispassionate view of homoeopathy, since any admission of virtue in homoeopathy was, and is, equivalent to criticizing medical "science."

In every country the adoption of homoeopathy by a sizable number of practitioners has split the medical profession into two irreconcilable groups. In the United States the formation of the American Institute of Homoeopathy in 1844 was the direct cause of the founding of the American Medical Association two years later. For sixty years the AMA was vehemently hostile to the homoeopaths. Regardless of the fact that many of the latter had graduated from Harvard, Dartmouth, Pennsylvania, and other leading medical schools, they were refused admittance to the orthodox medical societies. Professional consultation with a homoeopath was punished by ostracism and expulsion from these same medical societies.

These measures were not sufficient, however, to arrest the growth of homoeopathy, and during the latter half of the nineteenth century it was extremely widespread in New England, the Middle Atlantic states, and the Midwest. Being identified with New England transcendentalism, the doctrine made little headway in the South until the homoeopathic record in the 1878 yellow fever epidemic led to the conversion of many patients and physicians. Homoeopathy also had strongholds in Missouri, Iowa, Minnesota, and California, and individual practitioners could be found in every state and territory.

In 1890 there were about 14,000 homoeopaths in the country, as against about 85,000 "regular" physicians. In the areas of homoeopathy's greatest popularity, however, the proportion of homoeopathic physicians to regular ones was higher—perhaps one to four or one to five. Furthermore, it was admitted on all sides that the social, intellectual, political, and business elite of every community patronized the homoeopaths. Hence the power of the school was greater than its relatively small number of practitioners would indicate.

The AMA and its spokesmen viewed homoeopathy as a substantial threat to regular medicine all through the latter half of the nineteenth century. The existence of this threat spurred the production of a large body of polemical literature designed to prevent physicians from taking up this new doctrine and to win the homoeopathic patients back to medical orthodoxy.

The "medical education controversy" of the 1840's, which underlay the formation of the AMA, was actually a controversy over the cause of the defection of so many physicians to homoeopathy. The blame for this was ultimately laid at the door of American medical education.

The polemics continued until the end of the century and beyond, always stressing the homoeopath's alleged skill at ingratiating himself with his patients by his careful physical examination and his willingness to listen to a long recital of symptoms. Any cures were ascribed to the power of suggestion or to the natural recuperative potential of the organism. As the "regulars" gradually relinquished massive bloodletting and "heroic" quantities of medicines in the 1860's and 1870's, they began to admit that the homoeopathic "placebos" may have had some justification two or three decades earlier but also made plain that patients now had no further reasons for adhering to this system. Those who persisted (and the numbers of homoeopathic physicians and patients increased steadily up into the early 1900's) were characterized in the same terms as before.

The verbal warfare against homoeopathy continued until well into the twentieth century, even though these physicians were officially admitted into the regular medical societies in 1903 (on the condition that they cease calling themselves "homoeopaths" and cease proselytizing for homoeopathy!!), and the only reason it died down in the 1930's and 1940's was that the few homoeopaths remaining in practice in this country were too small a target to be worth the trouble.

However, orthodox medicine is still sensitive on this score and still ambivalent. In the 1920's the editor of the

AMA *Journal* wrote a book devoted, in part, to an "expose" of the homoeopathic doctrines which by that time had already been in the public domain for about 120 years. And even though most homoeopaths today are members of the AMA, a homoeopathic exhibit at the 1957 Cincinnati Centennial Medical Exhibition was closed down by agents of the AMA Bureau of Investigation, sent from Chicago for that specific purpose, who declared that the homoeopathic exhibit was "obnoxious and subversive."

Although the spokesmen for orthodox medicine and its organizations were willing to castigate both the homoeopathic patients and their physicians on the various scores mentioned above, they never conducted a controlled and supervised investigation of the merits of this system. The American Institute of Homoeopathy in 1912 offered to participate in such an investigation, but its offer was refused by the AMA. Individual allopathic physicians have investigated homoeopathy on their own, and the result in many cases has been their adoption of homoeopathy (nearly all the leading figures in American homoeopathy have been allopathic converts), but the allopathic organizations have never seen fit to take the relatively simple step of running a clinical test of homoeopathy—which might have resolved the issues between the two doctrines or at least have clarified some of the claims.

The arguments of the allopaths against homoeopathy have always been of a strongly *a priori* nature. It has been alleged, in particular, that such small doses of medicine "could not" possibly have the effects attributed to them. Hahnemann is said to have been influenced by German Romanticism (which is undoubtedly true). These arguments are apparently taken as proof positive that the homoeopathic practice is only a nullity, the systematic administration of placebos, etc.

It is generally accepted in scientific discourse, however, that facts come before theory. What is called "scientific method" is a technique for (among other things) reaching agreement on certain facts. Once there is general acceptance of the facts, the theory behind the facts can then be discussed. The essential fact to be ascertained about homoeopathy is whether or not these physicians can make their sick patients well by following the homoeopathic method. But decade after decade allopathic commentators have studiously refrained from verifying this one all-important fact. There are a number of homoeopaths in practice in the United States today, and it would not be difficult to find one and observe him (or her) in action. Then these writers would be better placed to judge the validity of their theoretical criticisms of homoeopathy.

Unfortunately, the condemnation of homoeopathy on *a priori* grounds is an ingrained tradition. Medical orthodoxy, which prides itself on being receptive to everything new and on accepting or condemning only on the basis of experience, has not followed its own prescription in the case of homoeopathy. It has never attempted to ascertain the therapeutic facts and has always condemned homoeopathy for its failure to conform to what orthodox doctrine currently views as "scientific."

But the facts are there for all to see. Aside from the existence of many thousands of homoeopathic physicians in practice in the mid-twentieth century in most countries of the world, who are able to compete perfectly successfully with the most recent discoveries of orthodox medicine, the historical record presents a strong *prima facie* case in favor of homoeopathy.

The standard description of the homoeopathic patient as a neurotic middle-aged maiden lady whose fancies were tickled by the attentiveness of the homoeopathic physician has no counterpart in life. This picture, painted in the 1840's by Oliver Wendell Holmes, and echoed by most commentators since that time, is pure fiction.

The homoeopathic method made its first pronounced impact on American and European thought during the cholera epidemic of 1832 when, by the accounts of all observers, the homoeopaths had a far higher recovery rate than the regular physicians (in Paris, for example, during this epidemic, the price of the homoeopathic medicine for cholera increased 100-fold). Other epidemic diseases in which homoeopathic practitioners distinguished themselves were scarlet fever, dysentery, meningitis, and yellow fever. The nineteenth-century homoeopathic records are full of cases of the successful treatment of these diseases. Homoeopaths were particularly successful in the illnesses of children. Furthermore, the typical homoeopathic physician of those days was a small-town practitioner who spent his whole life with a relatively unchanging group of families for whom he was the only doctor. Is it to be seriously contemplated that he made his reputation and kept his patients decade after decade, treating successfully all the diseases of infants and farm animals as well as those of his normal clientele, merely by power of suggestion? While there were certainly many cases in homoeopathic, as in orthodox, practice where the mere presence of the physician and an encouraging word were sufficient to bring about a recovery, anyone at all familiar with the history of nineteenth-century epidemiology will know that in thousands and millions of cases the only treatment was by the correct medicine. Unless the homoeopaths had had effective forms of medication, they could never have succeeded in making a place for themselves on the medical scene.

Perhaps the best evidence of the efficacy of the homoeopathic medicines is that many were subsequently taken over by the orthodox physicians. Many of these same medicines are still used in the day-to-day practice of the orthodox school, the best example being nitroglycerine for certain heart conditions. This substance was first used in angina pectoris and other heart conditions in the early 1850's by Constantine Hering (1800-1880), who is known as the father of American homoeopathy for his many therapeutic and other contributions. Hering published his results in 1857, and the first mention of this use of nitroglycerine in an allopathic work came only in 1882.

Even the major revolution in therapeutics of the late nineteenth century, effected by Pasteur, was only a further application of the fundamental homoeopathic principle of cure through similars. Pasteur maintained that he derived the idea of vaccination against rabies and other diseases from the work of Edward Jenner in smallpox, but it is hard to believe that he was unaware of the existence of several hundred homoeopaths in France who were applying the same therapeutic technique on a more general scale.

\* \* \* \* \*

By now the reader will have appreciated the two points implicit in the previous discussion: (1) homoeopathy is a coherent and valid approach to therapeutics, and (2) its practitioners and patients consider it to be more effective than "scientific" (or "allopathic") medicine. Parenthetically it may be noted that in a period such as the present, when orthodox practice seems to be in a stage of overmedication and polypharmacy, homoeopathy possesses the additional advantage of avoiding the problem of "adverse reactions."

But these comments raise a series of additional questions. If homoeopathy is such a highly effective mode of therapy, why has it not been universally adopted? Why, in particular, has the number of homoeopaths in the United States declined since the latter decades of the nineteenth century? And, finally, is homoeopathy a scientific form of medical practice?

The first of these questions raises an argument which has been made against homoeopathy from the beginning. Even in the 1820's Hahnemann's opponents scoffed at him for failing to bring over the entire profession to his point of view. And today it still seems self-evident that the superior mode of therapy will inevitably elicit the support of the medical profession as a whole; hence the critics of homoeopathy continue to advance the same argument.

Like so many self-evident truths, however, this particular one is found upon closer examination to be less self-evident than at first appears. The possibility has to be admitted that a superior mode of practice can be rejected on grounds unrelated to its therapeutic potential. And it is not difficult to demonstrate that the ordinary physician would have cogent grounds for rejecting the homoeopathic system, regardless of its therapeutic efficacy.

We have emphasized that the orthodox medical profession, headed by the AMA, adopted a decidedly hostile attitude toward homoeopathy shortly after the doctrine's introduction into the United States. A wall was erected between homoeopathy and allopathy, and the practice of homoeopathy, or consultation with homoeopaths, was absolutely forbidden by the Code of Ethics. Homoeopaths were classified as quacks—along with Thomsonians, herb doctors, and run-of-the-mill abortionists.

Many were the physicians expelled from their medical societies for violating this "ethical" rule.

The very severe professional consequences of defection to homoeopathy to some extent explain why it did not make greater inroads into the ranks of American allopathy. It took a very strong-minded and self-reliant physician to leap from the familiar into the unknown.

But this is not the whole story. The real question is: why have orthodox practitioners at all times felt an instinctive aversion to the homoeopathic tenets? To understand this aversion one must first grasp the theoretical structure of the homoeopathic doctrine.

The fundamental homoeopathic tenet that cure is through "similars" means that the remedy for any case of disease or illness is the substance which—when administered systematically to a healthy person—yields precisely the symptom-pattern of the given case. Before any substance can be used as a homoeopathic remedy it must be administered to healthy persons (known as "proving" it, from the German *Pruefung*). Comprehensive records are kept of the results of these provings. The homoeopathic works on materia medica give many pages of symptoms for each of the hundreds of medicines commonly used in homoeopathic practice. Constantine Hering's *Guiding Symptoms of Our Materia Medica*, for instance, comprises ten volumes of 500 pages each.

Thus when the homoeopath seeks the remedy whose symptomatology is precisely similar to the symptoms of the patient before him, he must isolate one single remedy from the 1500-odd remedies in the homoeopathic materia medica. This demands a very fine and subtle observation of the patient's symptoms, including many which would be entirely overlooked in allopathic practice. It also demands a very precise matching of the patient's symptoms with those in the books. Many remedies have roughly similar symptomatologies, but only the one most similar remedy will act curatively in the given case. Experience has shown that the incorrectly selected remedy will usually have no effect at all on the patient or, at the most, will alter his symptoms without acting curatively.

Homoeopathic prescribing demands both time and intellectual labor, and this system is hence out of step with the socio-economic determinants of modern medical practice. Today the allopathic physician strives to spend less and less time with each patient and to allocate as much as possible of his work to nurses and other para-medical personnel. In this way many can see 40 to 50 patients a day, spending from 8 to 12 minutes with each patient. This trend is furthered by the modern development of allopathic pharmacology, with its stress on "broad-spectrum" drugs—meaning ones which can be used in a multitude of different disease states. The use of such drugs cuts down greatly on the physician's task of selecting a suitable remedy.

The trend in orthodox medical practice toward reducing the work load on the physician, and thus maximizing his income, started in the late nineteenth century with the rise of specialization. It was aided by the reduction in the number of medical schools, and of medical graduates, which followed upon the adoption of the recommendations in the Flexner Report (1910). Thereafter the country saw a decline in the total number of physicians and a consequent increase in the number of patients handled by each. The homoeopaths, who had previously enjoyed generally higher incomes than the regular physicians, now found that they could earn more money for less work in orthodox practice. Many switched to allopathy and reserved homoeopathic treatment for their families and a few favored patients. The reason for the switch was economic and not therapeutic.

The physician-patient ratio today is the lowest in American history, and economic forces thus continue to favor allopathic practice. There are many signs, however, of a popular revolt against this practice, comparable to the revolt of the 1830's and 1840's which ensconced homoeopathy on the American medical scene. Patients instinctively feel that no doctor can do a good job in 8 to 12 minutes. The broad-spectrum drugs, which so greatly simplify the physician's work because of their non-specific impact on pathological processes, often have a less than beneficial impact on the patient's overall health. Drugs of such indiscriminate effect are bound to produce consequences different from those anticipated. These "side-effects" (which are no less direct than any other effects of the medicine) have come increasingly to bedevil orthodox practice, and no solution is in sight.

Consequently, more and more patients are turning to homoeopathy. These physicians have more work than they can

9

easily handle, and the future of American homoeopathy is brighter today than it has been for decades.

The further spread of homoeopathy among physicians, however, is still seriously hampered by the unfamiliarity of the homoeopathic doctrine and the instinctive antipathy to it of most physicians who have received orthodox medical training. This antipathy is due in large part to the tendency of the homoeopathic doctrine to slight the pathological indications of disease in favor of the symptoms. One of the axioms of orthodox medical thought since Galen has been that pathology takes precedence over symptoms, and the school-trained physician of today can with difficulty bring himself to agree with the homoeopathic stress on the symptoms.

While the homoeopaths do not altogether ignore pathology, they rely on the symptoms for selecting the remedy. The remedies have been proven for their sense-perceptible symptoms alone, and these must be the physician's guide to treatment. This is not to be confused with "symptomatic" treatment in orthodox practice. The homoeopaths claim that when the patient receives the one single remedy whose symptomatology most perfectly matches his own symptoms, the whole disease—root, cause, and all—is entirely removed.

That this procedure is indeed reliable can be seen by the longevity of the homoeopathic procedures. Homoeopaths have always felt that pathological data are basically speculative and changeable, and for that reason are not a reliable basis for therapy. Symptoms, however, are unchanging. Observations made 150 years ago are still true today. Cases published in the 1830's still yield valuable information. A science based on the accurate and thorough observation of symptoms is long-lasting.

A final objection often made to homoeopathy is that it is "unscientific." Indeed, if the orthodox medical procedures are taken as scientific, then homoeopathy must be unscientific by very definition. But the homoeopaths have always denied that allopathy is scientific and have claimed instead that homoeopathy is the only scientific therapeutics.

How are we to evaluate the respective claims of the two systems to scientific status?

This task is made difficult by the ambivalence of allopathic medicine toward its own scientific basis. The modern orthodox physician will say that the scientific part of his system of practice derives from its precision in the observation and measurement of certain physiological and pathological phenomena. When it comes to the prescribing of a medicine or a mode of therapy, however, this same physician will admit that science stops and the physician's experience, intuition, or "sixth sense" takes over.

In any case, modern regular medicine is admittedly not scientific in its most important aspect—the prescription of the remedy. Homoeopathy, on the other hand, is strong where allopathy is weak and apparently weak where allopathy is strong. If we take the latter point first, homoeopathy's apparent weakness consists in its reliance on symptomatic data for evidence about the patient's health and the course of his disease. Its strength lies in the usually unambiguous indication of the remedy. A complete picture of the patient's symptoms will, in nine cases out of ten, point to one remedy and one only. Confronted with a given symptom-pattern, a group of homoeopaths will all prescribe the same remedy.

Thus what makes homoeopathy scientific, in the opinion of its practitioners, is the rigor of its method. The homoeopathic method is very precise, and the practice of this form of therapeutics is a demanding discipline. When criticized for basing their method upon the non-quantifiable and non-measurable symptoms, and thus allegedly rejecting precise techniques for observing and measuring the phenomena of disease and health, the homoeopaths reply that the precisely observed symptom is still the most accurate measure of disease and health. The allopathic techniques—sedimentation rates, electrocardiograms, blood counts, and the like—are all too crude and indiscriminate for the homoeopathic taste. They fail to make the precise distinctions among cases which are possible in homoeopathy.

It must be admitted in favor of the homoeopathic position that the difference between an amorphous body of data and a science is that the data in the latter are developed and organized into a coherent whole through application of a method. "Scientific method" is a set of integrated procedures

11

applied to the organization and study of the phenomena of the particular science. This is done by formulating hypotheses and testing them against the facts of experience.

Homoeopathy possesses its hypothesis—the doctrine of similars—and its method, the proving of remedies on the healthy and their administration to the sick on the basis of symptom-similarity. Ordinary "scientific" medicine possesses neither an all-encompassing hypothesis upon which therapy may be based nor a generally applicable method for ascertaining the curative remedy. Every time a homoeopath administers a medicine to a patient he is performing an experiment which tests the truth of his hypothesis. Every time the patient recovers, the experiment can be considered a success, and one more piece of evidence is accumulated in favor of the truth of the doctrine of similars.

Discussion of this point could be prolonged indefinitely, since it is both complex in itself and made more so by the ambiguity of orthodox medicine about its own scientific basis. Enough has been said to show that a good case can be made for the scientific standing of homoeopathy. That it should have remained unchanged for 180 years is seen by these physicians as further evidence of its scientific nature, since a true science is cumulative. New information from the provings of new substances can be integrated into the existing doctrine without nullifying all that has gone before—in decided contrast to orthodox medicine where new discoveries often make obsolete most of the previously accepted knowledge and where future discoveries will doubtless vitiate most of what is today accepted as "scientific" truth.

In the discussion of the scientific nature of homoeopathy, as in so much else connected with this school of practice, disagreement in theory is caused by disagreement over the facts. If it were generally conceded that homoeopaths do indeed cure their patients systematically by following procedures based upon the doctrine of similars, it would be difficult indeed to call this doctrine unscientific. For what can a scientific medicine be, other than a method for curing people? This point is occasionally forgotten in orthodox medicine, which seems at times to seek the "advancement of medical science" as an end in itself. But it is never forgotten by the homoeopaths for whom the therapeutic part of medicine is the methodical—hence scientific—part, to which the rest must be subordinate.

Since the present incomprehension of homoeopathy is rooted in ignorance of the relevant facts, the following pages set forth a series of facts which will make homoeopathic theory and practice more accessible to the public generally, and especially to persons with some medical training.

# Chapter One
# Homoeopathy's Position in the World Today

Before embarking on an analysis of homoeopathy as a science, the reader should know something about the social and economic dimensions of this unusual medical phenomenon.

Although Germany was its birthplace, homoeopathy made its way in 1825 to the United States — the country upon which it would have the most profound impact. Within a few decades an independent homoeopathic profession had come into existence there, with separate examining and licensing boards and its own system of medical schools and hospitals.

Homoeopathic medical education was recognized on all sides as the equal of allopathic, and the two systems of practice were treated as equals under the federal and state law. As late as 1938 the Food, Drug and Cosmetic Act recognized the *United States Homoeopathic Pharmacopoeia* as the legal equivalent of the (allopathic) *United States Pharmacopoeia*.

And today, since the separate homoeopathic medical schools and licensing boards have disappeared, the homoeopathic M.D. must attend the ordinary medical schools and pass the same qualifying and licensing examinations as all other physicians.

While this therapeutic method is practiced by only a minority of physicians, in the United States and elsewhere, it is experiencing a resurgence in all countries. Younger physicians are attracted to it not only for its therapeutic efficacy but also because of the absence of any problem with the "side effects," "adverse reactions," and iatrogenic diseases which seem to be inevitable concomitants of allopathic medicine.

In many countries steps have been taken to strengthen homoeopathy's legal position. The most recent instance is the new Drug Law in the German Federal Republic (1978) which establishes a separate register for homoeopathic drugs and thus affords them legal protection. In England the Parliament adopted the Faculty of Homoeopathy Act in 1950. incorporating the faculty of the Royal London Homoeopathic Hospital and empowering it to issue diplomas of competence in homoeopathy; the National Health Service reimburses homoeopathic physicians for treatment. In France the official pharmacopoeia has a separate section for homoeopathic medicines. The U.S.S.R., Rumania, and other countries of Eastern Europe give state support to homoeopathic clinics. In Pakistan the government recognized homoeopathy officially in 1965 and has allocated funds for establishing homoeopathic colleges; homoeopathic prescriptions are also reimbursed under the national health service. India has a large number of homoeopathic colleges, many of which are supported by the state governments or the federal government. In 1970 the government of Sri Lanka (Ceylon) passed a homoeopathy bill which accorded official recognition to this method of practice. Mexico has several homoeopathic medical schools, both public and private, of which the leading one is the Escuela Nacional de Medicina Homoeopática. The Greek government has recently taken an interest in homoeopathy, and the 31st International Homoeopathic Congress (1976) was held in Athens under the auspices of the Greek Ministry of Culture and Science. In Brazil the government-financed Federal Medical School has a professor of clinical homoeopathy.

And yet, despite the evidence of worldwide interest in homoeopathy and the official support given to this method of practice in a number of countries, it still remains largely a mystery to the physicians who do not employ it themselves.

This short treatise aims to present the principles of homoeopathy in a way which will be intelligible to allopathic physicians and medical students trained in allopathic medical schools. Thus the ensuing discussion is largely in the language, and based on the concepts, of allopathic medicine.

16

After a statement of homoeopathic principles, there follows a series of sections exemplifying these principles in terms of allopathic concepts, investigations, and practices. Another section discusses homoeopathic clinical experience. And the Conclusion presents an overall contrast between homoeopathy and allopathy with particular reference to the principles of scientific method.

# Chapter Two
# The Doctrinal Basis of Homoeopathic Practice

Homoeopathy differs from allopathy in possessing a precise set of principles governing diagnosis and treatment. The physician who does not follow these principles more or less accurately cannot be said to practice homoeopathy, even though he may on occasion employ homoeopathic medicines.

An American physician, Ian Stevenson, wrote in 1949 that "the basic laws of health and disease" have not yet been disclosed. Indeed, "the search for these laws has hardly begun. No discipline can claim a greater array of equipment by which its research is carried on, yet none is inferior to medicine in organizing its knowledge into coherent principles." [1]

This critique of allopathic medicine is a useful point at which to commence an examination of homoeopathy — which is the mirror image of the above picture, having always insisted on the necessity of practicing medicine guided by a set of principles of disease and health. Homoeopathy has always adhered to a set of assumptions about the functioning of the human organism in health and disease, the nature of its relationship to the external world, and the effects of the medicines used to treat disease. Since these assumptions are quite precise, the rules of homoeopathic practice are also precise.

Thus the first point to be borne in mind is that homoeopathy consists of a body of principles forming a coherent whole. These principles have been tested in practice for about 180 years, and the homoeopathic physicians feel that their scientific validity has been conclusively demonstrated.

While the application of these principles has expanded somewhat from decade to decade with the entry of new medicinal substances into homoeopathic practice, the principles themselves have not altered.

The purpose of these principles, and of the rules of practice emanating from them, is to enable the physician to discover for each sick person the medicinal substance which most closely meets his needs.

Thus homoeopathy is a system of pharmacological medicine, a set of rules for administering specially prepared drugs to sick people and thereby making them well. While surgery, diet, exercise, etc. are very important for health and are often recommended by the homoeopathic physician, they have nothing to do with the homoeopathic doctrine itself which is a set of rules for administering drugs.

Strict adherence to these rules enables the conscientious and painstaking physician to prescribe for each patient the precise medicine which will act curatively in his case.


Homoeopathy views the living organism as unceasingly reacting to its environment, attempting to ward off danger and repair damage. Thus, what is called "sickness" actually represents the organism's striving after health. The patient's symptoms are not the impact of some morbific stimulus on his organism but are the *reaction* of the organism to the morbific stimulus.

One corollary of this assumption is that all illness is "general" — representing the curative effort of the whole body. Homoeopathy does not recognize the existence of "local" illness. It does not admit that several such "local" illnesses can coexist in the body. Illness is always "general," and the patient can never suffer from more than one illness at a time, however many local manifestations this one illness may yield.

A second corollary is that the symptoms, however painful and undesirable, are beneficial phenomena, since they

19

indicate the pathway taken by the organism in its attempt to restore health.

A third corollary is that the symptoms are more important for diagnosis and treatment than are the structural or material alterations in the organism. This is because symptoms are chronologically prior to structural changes and lead the way to the structural changes.

Hence the homoeopathic physician sees his task as promoting the curative effort of the organism indicated by the symptoms. The homoeopathic therapeutic doctrine shows him how to assist the organism in this self-healing effort. It is a *set of rules* enabling him to select the medicine which, when administered to the sick person, will stimulate his self-healing effort along the lines already adopted.

The first of these rules is that the medicine must be prescribed according to the "law of similars" — meaning that the appropriate remedy for each sick person is the substance which would give rise to precisely his set of symptoms if administered to a healthy person.

The concept of treating with "similars" is very ancient and was resurrected in the early nineteenth century by Edward Jenner's use of cowpox vaccination as a preventive of smallpox. The "similar" cowpox was seen to confer immunity against smallpox. Later in the century Pasteur developed a vaccine against rabies which was made from the dried spinal cords of rabbits dead of rabies — thus, also a "similar." In the twentieth century immunization techniques have been developed for yellow fever, plague, poliomyelitis, and other diseases: the principle of treatment by "similars" received extensive application.

In the above instances the "similarity" is between the causal agents of the diseases: rabies in rabbits, rabies in man; cowpox and smallpox; polio in monkeys, polio in man, etc. Homoeopathy investigated this interpretation of "similarity" in the 1830's but rejected it in favor of similarity, not of cause, but of *symptom*.

To clarify, the powers of medicines are discovered in the homoeopathic school by administering these medicines in very small quantities to healthy persons for an extended period of time — weeks or months. This is called "proving" the medicine, from the German word, *Pruefung*, meaning "test" or "trial." Every substance in the world — animal, vegetable, or mineral — produces its own specific and peculiar set of symptoms when administered systematically to healthy persons. The literature of the homoeopathic school consists of such collections of the symptoms of about 1500 medicines.

Hahnemann was led to his discovery of the rules of homoeopathy by his curiosity about the reason for the curative effect of quinine in malaria. He experimented on himself, taking quinine in moderate doses for a period of time, and found that he manifested the typical symptoms of an attack of malaria. From this he concluded that quinine is curative in malaria through its ability to generate the typical symptoms of this disease.

The homoeopathic medicines include many substances used traditionally in Western medicine — *Belladonna, Aconitum napellus, Colchicum, Camphor, Veratrum, Mercury, Sulphur, Digitalis, Nitroglycerine, Arsenic, Aurum* (gold), *Plumbum* (lead), *Secale cornutum* (ergot), etc. (many of which are still in use today), but to them have been added hundreds more, including some — such as silica or sodium chloride (table salt) — which have not been regarded by allopathy as possessing therapeutic powers.

The provings of these substances yield groups of symptoms which define precisely how the healthy organism reacts to the specific stimulus represented by each such substance. And these proving-symptoms thereby indicate precisely how the given substance is to be used for treatment. Since the symptoms of the sick person represent his curative reaction to the morbific stimulus, the most effective way to cure him will necessarily be through prescribing the substance which intensifies these curative symptoms.

When confronted with a sick person, therefore, the homoeopathic physician first undertakes to elicit from him all his symptoms. This is a lengthy and complex process, requiring more time and effort than the anamnesis performed by the non-homoeopathic physician. He will inquire into the patient's past history, and perhaps the medical history of his parents and siblings, to obtain a full picture of his medical background.

Addendum II, written by James Tyler Kent (1849-1916) — the greatest American-born homoeopathic physician, shows how this questioning is done. While a physician will not pose all these questions in any one case, Kent's exposition reveals the detail which homoeopathy demands if a comprehensive picture of the patient's ailments is to be obtained.

Then the physician investigates the literature of the provings to ascertain precisely which substance produces a set of symptoms identical with that of the patient. This is the indicated remedy because it will intensify the incipient healing process. The patient's symptoms represent the commencement of this healing process, and the medicine generating these symptoms is the one which helps carry through the healing process to cure (or to the next stage of recovery).

The use of one single remedy at a time is preferred, and considered better homoeopathy. By finding the one remedy whose symptoms match the totality of the patient's symptoms, the homoeopathic physician is prescribing the one remedy which meets the needs of the patient's whole organism. This makes homoeopathy a holistic mode of practice.

Although the homoeopathic physician is guided by the patient's symptoms, he is not prescribing "symptomatically." He treats, not the patient's symptoms, but his whole organism — whose needs are made manifest through the totality of his symptoms.

The homoeopathic physician must use the "minimum dose." The reason for this rule is easy to understand. When medicines are employed according to the principle of similars, a large dose will tend to exacerbate the patient's existing symptom-pattern. Only a "minimum dose" will effect cure without a severe aggravation of the patient's symptoms.

Thus it is customary in homoeopathy to talk of Hahnemann's three rules of prescribing: (1) strict adherence to the law of similars, (2) the single remedy, and (3) the minimum dose.

It must be confessed, however, that the meaning of "minimum" in this context is ambiguous in view of the homoeopathic principle that medicines become more powerful with greater dilution. Hahnemann himself lowered his doses to thousandths and millionths of a grain, causing allopathic physicians in the nineteenth century to scoff at homoeopathy's supposed use of placebos. It was only with the twentieth century's discovery of hormones and other substances which are also effective in microscopically small quantities that allopathic physicians have to some extent ceased deriding the homoeopathic "high dilutions." (Addendum I presents the typical levels of dilution employed in homoeopathic pharmacology).

Hahnemann claimed that these high dilutions are effective because the sick person is ultrasensitive to the action of the similar remedy. He wrote, as early as 1810, that "there are patients whose impressionibility, compared to that of unsusceptible ones, is in the ratio of 1000 to 1."

This ultrasensitivity of the sick person to the "similar," together with the stimulant effect of the similar remedy on the reactive process in the organism, means that the correct homoeopathic prescription is often followed by a momentary aggravation of the symptoms.

The homoeopathic use of the small dose may be viewed from a different angle. Hahnemann discovered that any medicinal substance gives rise initially to a set of "primary" symptoms, followed in time by a different set of "secondary" symptoms more or less the "opposite" of the "primary" symptoms. If a large dose is used, the "primary" symptoms are prominent, and the "secondary" ones (representing the reaction of the organism) are weak. If the dose is small, the "primary" symptoms are less apparent, and only the "secondary" ones appear. Thus it is customary to speak of the "opposite" effects of large and small doses.

In the light of this discussion, the homoeopathic small dose is seen to be the one which, without initially depressing the organism, stimulates its reactive healing power.

The only major addition to Hahnemann's original doctrine is known as Hering's Law in honor of its discoverer, Constantine Hering (1800-1880) of Philadelphia — the intellectual leader of the nineteenth-century American homoeopathic school.

Hering's Law holds that as a disease passes from an acute to a chronic form the symptoms move from the surface of the body to the interior, from the lower part of the body to the upper, and from the less vital organs to the more vital. This is also true, in part, for the movement of symptoms in acute disease. Under correct homoeopathic treatment this movement is reversed, and the symptoms will then move from the more vital organs to the less vital, from the upper part of the body to the lower, and from the interior to the skin. Furthermore, they will disappear in the reverse order of their appearance.

An important corollary of Hering's Law, and also of the homoeopathic principle that all illness is general, is that so-called "mental" illness is only an extreme form of a general morbific process — one whose symptoms have penetrated: (1) deep inside the body, (2) high up in the body, and (3) to one of the most vital organs, the brain. All disease processes have a mental aspect (mental symptoms) as well as a somatic one. So-called "mental" illness is only a morbific process in which the mental aspects are more prominent than the somatic ones. Since the homoeopathic provings all yield mental as well as somatic symptoms, "mental" illnesses are treated in homoeopathy according to the same method that is used to treat "physical" illness.

Another very important corollary of Hering's Law is that skin eruptions and skin diseases are to be regarded as very positive manifestations, signs of passage of the illness from the inside of the body to the outside. Hence, topical applications are never used in homoeopathy for the treatment of so-called "skin diseases," as such applications are considered to act suppressively, rooting the illness into the organism and causing it to assume a chronic form.

Hering's Law is extremely important for homoeopathic practice since it outlines the natural course which must be followed by morbific and curative processes. As Hering himself stated: "Only such patients remain well and are really cured who have been rid of their symptoms in the reverse order of their development." The physician is not justified in attempting short cuts. He must respect the stages of illness. He can only prescribe on the basis of the symptoms presenting during the given stage, and he hopes that the prescribed remedy will move the disease in the direction of cure.

It follows that failure to respect the natural process of illness and recovery will cause harm to the patient. Specifically, the homoeopathic school has found from experience that allopathic treatment of acute illness may engraft on the patient an incurable chronic illness.

This homoeopathic interpretation of chronic disease has definite implications for the attitude to be taken to the epidemic of chronic disease in modern industrial societies.

From the preceding discussion we may isolate eight elements of homoeopathic doctrine in support of which evidence may be marshalled from the non-homoeopathic literature:

—The reactivity of the organism to external stimuli; disease as an expression of the adaptive effort of the whole organism; priority of symptomatic changes over structural or pathological changes.

—The biphasal action of medicines.

—The provings.

—Ultrasensitivity of the organism to the similar medicine; aggravation.

—The infinitesimal dose; homoeopathic rejection of the monotonicity rule.

—The single remedy.

—The law of similars.

—Hering's Law and chronic disease.

These eight elements of doctrine are discussed in the eight sections which follow.

# Chapter Three
# Symptoms As Positive Phenomena

**(a) The Organism's Reactivity to External Stimuli**

The capacity of the organism to respond in a variety of ways, and at different levels, to environmental stimuli is a commonplace of medicine. The adjustment and adaptation of the organism to its environment are mediated through the endocrine and nervous systems and undoubtedly through other modes of dynamic adjustment still unknown to medical science and unexplained by it. S. Solis-Cohen wrote: "life is a continuous adjustment of internal relations to external relations . . . living beings maintain a moving equilibrium in harmony with their changing environment by automatically effecting internal changes to counterbalance external ones. The ability to effect such counterbalancing adjustments promptly and adequately constitutes health." [2] Hans Selye's numerous writings on "stress" assume the existence of this purposive reactive capacity of the organism and its parts: "stress responses are purposeful homeostatic reactions." [3] "stress is defined as the nonspecific response of the body to any demand," [4] "even a single cell can respond in qualitatively different (specific or non-specific) ways." [5]

Selye emphasizes that the stress reaction — which he also calls the "general adaptation syndrome" — is largely independent of the nervous system and in some way innate to the body's tissues: it can be produced in plants (which do not have a nervous system), in a limb from which the nerves have been removed, and even in a cell culture grown outside the body.[6]

At some point the interplay between organism and environment begins to work against the organism; the balance is tipped in favor of the environment and against the living body. Here the symptoms of health are transformed into what we regard as the symptoms of disease, painful manifestations which are disagreeable to the sufferer. However, this state of "ill-health" is not qualitatively different from the state of health, being merely a quantitative move along the spectrum of the interaction between organism and environment. Many allopathic authorities have maintained that "pathology" does not differ qualitatively from "physiology" and that "disease" is only a continuation of processes occurring during the state of "health." W. H. Perkins wrote in 1938:

> Every function can be stressed beyond the limits of its accepted normal; when this is so, the altered function is called abnormal, and the evidence of it is pathology. In so doing, an arbitrary indefinite line has been created between the two states, which is variably called the "borderline of disease," the "limit of safety," the "limit of tolerance," or the "normal limit" . . . it must be admitted that disease cannot accurately be defined.[7]

Karl Menninger stated in 1948:

> I believe that clinicians have come to think of disease more and more in terms of a disturbance in the total economics of the personality, a temporary overwhelming of the efforts of the organism to maintain a continuous internal and external adaptation to continuously changing relationships, threats, pressures, instinctual needs, and reality demands. . . . It is the imbalance, the organismic disequilibrium, which is the real pathology, and when that imbalance reaches a degree or duration that threatens the comfort or survival of the individual, it may be correctly denoted disease.[8]

A modern text proclaims:

> Disease syndromes are transient aspects of the reaction of the whole individual to his total environment . . . their occurrence is governed as much by the relation of the indi-

27

vidual to his social environment as by his random contact with specific etiologic factors. The effect of the stimulus depends in great degree not only on the type of stimulus but on the state of the individual and his response. Some adapt more readily than others. These data tell us how little we really know of the underlying factors producing host reactions.[9]

And Selye writes:

Textbooks usually define health as the absence of disease, and vice-versa. These "definitions" rest upon the assumption that the two conditions are the opposites of each other. Is this really so? Are they not rather different only in degree and in the position of vital phenomena proceeding within time-space?[10]

Disease is not mere surrender to attack but also fight for health; unless there is a fight there is no disease.[11]

Disease is not just suffering, but a fight to maintain the homeostatic balance of our tissues, despite damage.[12]

Even diseases associated with bacteria, viruses, and other microorganisms depend to a large, and still unclear, extent on the reactivity or susceptibility of the organism. Zinsser wrote that pathogenic microorganisms may reside in the body for extended periods without producing manifest disease: "thus, perfectly normal individuals may on occasion harbor organisms of the latter variety over varying periods of time."[13] More recently Rene Dubos has observed:

The ability of microorganisms to produce pathologic changes is under the influence of large biologic forces as yet poorly understood . . . the mechanism through which microbial agents reach their potential victims and elicit pathologic reactions are known in their broad outline, but this knowledge has not yet been reconciled with the fact — now well established — that extremely virulent pathogens are often present in the tissues of normal individuals, who exhibit neither signs nor symptoms of disease. Today, the most puzzling problem of medical microbiology is no longer: "How do microorganisms cause disease?" but rather, "Why do pathogens so often fail to cause disease after they have become established in the tissues?" Curiously enough, this question is rarely asked and even more rarely submitted to experimental analysis.[14]

This same interpretation of disease and health is found in the science of allergology. Warren T. Vaughan, a leading allergist of the 1930's, wrote that the allergic state is merely a more extreme manifestation of a condition found in the healthy individual: "There is no fundamental difference between the allergic and the so-called non-allergic individual. The response of the allergic person differs from the non-allergic in degree, not in kind. . . . Allergy is not a pathologic state. It is a pathological exaggeration of a normal physiologic response."[15]

### (b) Disease as the Adaptive Effort of the Whole Organism

Homoeopathy maintains that all disease is general and denies the possibility of "local" disease or "local" treatment. The patient's symptoms represent the totality of his response to a given morbific stimulus (insult). Selye's "general adaptation syndrome" is the most striking modern expression of this idea:

I called this syndrome *general* because it is produced only by agents which have a general effect upon large portions of the body. I called it *adaptive* because it stimulates defense and thereby helps in the acquisition and maintenance of a state of inurement. I called it a *syndrome* because its individual manifestations are coordinated and even partly dependent upon each other.[16]

Other allopathic writers are ambiguous on this point, regarding some types of illnesses as "general" or systemic and others as "local":

The chronic inflammatory bowel diseases are incurable systemic diseases with the gut as their target organ.[17]

For more than 50 years research in cancer has been based on the concept that cancer is a disease of cells and therefore that the cause and cure of cancer are to be found within the cell. . . . Work of the past several decades has

29

demonstrated clearly that the central nervous system and the peripheral endocrine system are intricately involved in the organism's response to stress. ... This concept requires a new approach to the cancer problem — an approach which demands a study of the organism as a whole.[18]

Theories on the nature of cancer may be classified into two categories. One regards cancer strictly as a local phenomenon while the second looks at cancer as a local manifestation of a systemic process or disease. Although the first dominates current medical thought, the theories of immunological surveillance and of protovirus-oncogene implicitly assume cancer to represent a local manifestation of a systemic process or disease.[19]

Arteriosclerosis could be regarded as a prototype of a systemic disease. It presents itself clinically solely by its local manifestations, like myocardial infarction or stroke. These local manifestations may be followed by secondary systemic sequelae like congestive heart failure.[20]

From the homoeopathic point of view, allopathy here is often inconsistent since, even when a disease is classified as "systemic," treatment may be local. For example, cortisone enemas are sometimes used to treat ulcerative colitis (a "systemic disease with the gut as ... target organ").

If disease is seen as a reactive effort of the organism, it would seem logical to interpret the symptom as a manifestation of this reactive effort, i.e., as a positive and beneficial phenomenon, pointing the way to health. In allopathic medicine this interpretation of the symptom is encountered rather rarely:

The symptoms of bacterial disease express the effort made by tissues and humors to adapt themselves to the new conditions, to resist them, and to return to a normal state. ... Each tissue is capable of responding, at any moment of the unpredictable future, to all physico-chemical or chemical changes of the intraorganic medium in a manner consistent with the interests of the whole body.[21]

Most of the clinical symptoms of infectious disease are due to the reaction of the body.[22]

The mode of action of a pathogenic agent in the body of a suitable host is evidenced . . . principally by the symptomatic reaction on the part of the individual.[23]

Selye demonstrates that the symptoms of inflammation — heat, reddening, swelling, and pain — are part of the body's defense reaction, serving to limit and contain injury.[24]

But allopathy most commonly interprets the symptom as the sign of a morbific change or pathological alteration within the body; this, of course, is logically incompatible with the idea that "disease" is an expression of the organism's *reaction* to a morbific stimulus.[25]

A third interpretation seen sometimes in allopathic writings holds that symptoms are a mixture of the signs of pathological alteration and the signs of the body's reactive effort, i.e., "symptoms include phenomena of two opposite orders: a) those of derangement, and b) those of restorative adjustment or recovery . . . almost from the first they exist side by side . . . the physician must discriminate between the two orders of phenomena."[25] Selye writes: "reactions which tend to repair wear and tear are not strictly stress, but rather responses to stress. However, in practice it is rarely (if ever) possible to distinguish clearly between damage and repair."[26]

The idea that symptoms represent a beneficial reaction is encountered in the field of allergy. Warren T. Vaughan stated that "the allergic response is primarily a protective reaction," and gave the following justification:

When a noxious substance enters the nose, its removal is accomplished by sneezing and the secretion of mucus. The cough, smooth muscle spasm, and increased bronchial secretion of asthma may be looked upon as an attempt to remove a supposed foreign body. Asthma may develop for the first time in connection with a tumor growth in the lung. This is often true asthma and may be relieved by adrenalin or ephedrin. It represents a physiologic reaction, an attempt to remove a foreign body from the lungs. Prompt vomiting which sometimes follows the ingestion of an allergenic food is again a protective response, as is the hyperperistalsis and diarrhoea associated with mucous colitis which often follows the ingestion of an allergenic food which the stomach has not repelled. The serous exudation of a contact dermatitis represents an effort to wash away the noxious substance. Lichenification in chronic dermatitis indicates an effort to establish a protective thickening of the skin at the point of contact. Urticaria and angioneurotic edema which involve internal structures probably to nearly as great an extent as they do the visible integument manifest an effort to dilute the allergenic substance in the tissues, thus protecting the living cells.[27]

If this argument is followed a little further, the anaphylactic state is seen to be an extreme form of the protective condition represented by allergy:

There is no fundamental difference between clinical allergy and experimental anaphylaxis.[28]

It was and still is our opinion that the allergic reaction is an integral part of the specific immune response and represents an increased reaction capacity of the protective mechanism to contact with the invading organisms.[29]

Antibodies are not only produced as a defense mechanism against invading pathogenic organisms or their toxic products, but are the response of the host to the introduction of any kind of foreign antigenic material, especially foreign proteins. . . . Therefore, it becomes obvious that the production of antibodies is a general biologic phenomenon rather than a specialized mechanism designed to protect against infection. . . . Antibody production means not only protection but also hypersensitization, as revealed by experimental anaphylaxis in animals and asthma in man.[30]

### (c) Symptomatic Changes Prior to Structural or Pathological Changes

The idea that symptoms are chronologically prior to structural change or pathological alteration, and hence of more importance as diagnostic guides, is occasionally encountered in orthodox medical thought:

32

Symptoms are apt to appear some time before striking physical signs of disease are evident and before laboratory tests are useful in detecting disordered physiology.[31]

A patient's sore tongue and mouth may be the only grossly visible sign that he has nutritional deficiency disease. Yet he is sick in every cell of his body and, indeed, has been biochemically sick for a variable period of time (the prodromal period of the deficiency state) prior to the appearance of the first gross or microscopic lesion.[32]

# Chapter Four
# The Biphasal Action
# of Medicines

Interpreting the patient's symptoms as positive signs of reaction, Hahnemann logically concluded that cure would be brought about by any drug or medicinal substance which supported this reaction, and it was this which led him to the idea of cure through similars. The medicine which, in a healthy person, gives rise to precisely the symptom-pattern of the given patient is the medicine which will cure that patient.

But the concept of cure through similars has its complexities. Hahnemann discovered that any drug administered to a sick or healthy person gives rise to two successive symptom-patterns. The first, which he called the "primary" symptoms, may be taken as the immediate effect of the drug on the organism; the second, which Hahnemann called the "secondary" symptoms, may be regarded as the reaction of the organism to the immediate drug effect. The "secondary" symptoms are more or less the opposite of the "primary" symptoms.

Hahnemann found that the relationship between "primary" and "secondary" symptoms was to some extent a function of dose size. If a large dose was given to a patient, the primary symptoms were too violent, while the secondary reaction was also disordered. If a very small dose was given, the primary effect was minimal and was soon succeeded by the secondary one (disappearance of the patient's symptoms).

Because of this relationship to dose size, the biphasal action of medicines is often described as the "opposite" effect of small and large doses. But this is inaccurate, since the two sets of symptoms are present in all cases, the difference being in their relative strength and prominence.

Hahnemann decided that if the "primary" symptoms of the medicine, when administered to a healthy person, were identical with the symptoms of the sick patient, the "secondary" symptoms of the medicine would act to remove the patient's symptoms and thus restore him to health.

Hahnemann's discovery was taken up by conventional medicine in the late ninetenth century and expressed as the so-called Arndt-Schulz Law: "every drug has a stimulating effect in small doses, while larger doses inhibit, and much larger doses kill." It was further refined by the German physician, Karl Koetschau, in the 1920's as the "type effect hypothesis" which posits three typical effects of a medicinal drug, depending upon dose (see the following diagram):

1. with small doses a stimulant effect (the A curve),
2. with moderate doses an effect which is at first stimulant but then depressive, with the patient eventually returning to normal (the B curve), and
3. with large doses a very brief stimulant effect followed by a severely depressive effect leading to death (the C curve).

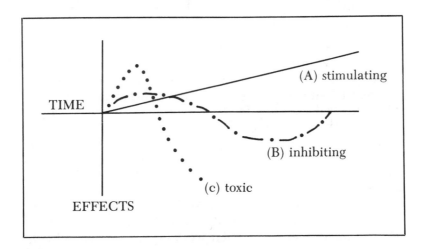

35

In this connection it is understood that the meaning of "large" and "small" doses will depend upon the medicine used. And with certain substances the reverse curves appear (the A curve, for example, will be a depression).[33]

In the early 1950's Joseph Wilder proposed a reformulation of the Arndt-Schulz and Koetschau rules. His Law of Initial Value reads as follows:

> Not only the intensity but also the direction of a response of a body function to any agent depend to a large degree on the initial level of that function at the start of the experiment. The higher this "initial level," the smaller is the response to function-raising, the greater is the response to function-depressing agents. At more extreme initial levels there is a progressive tendency to "no response" and to "paradoxic reactions," i.e., a reversal of the usual direction of the response.[34]

By the same token, the lower the "initial level," the greater the response to "function raising" agents and the less the response to "function depressing" ones.

Wilder noted that his proposed law contradicts common-sense opinion in medicine:

> It is necessary to emphasize that most investigators do not take the initial levels into account at all. If they do, they operate usually with the tacit assumption that the opposite of our law is true: e.g., that a hypertensive individual will respond to adrenalin with a higher rise in pressure than one who is normotensive.[35]

Thus, where the Arndt-Schulz and Koetschau rules were formulated in terms of the size of the pharmacological dose, Wilder's rule is expressed in terms of the varying sensitivity of different organisms to a given dose size: what is "small" for one individual may be "medium" for another and a "large" dose for a third, yielding different effects in each individual. In all cases, however, the phenomenon of interest is the "reversal of the usual direction of response," whether it is a function of change in dose size or of the altered sensitivity of the organism.

Selye gives an example of the Wilder Law of Initial Value: while excessive stimulation of a muscle can produce local inflammation, intense muscular work suppresses the ability of the overworked muscular tissue to become inflamed by local application of an irritant substance.[36]

Wilder observed in 1957 that few, if any, pharmacological investigations take the initial state of the organism into account even though this "is at least as important as the establishment of proper controls." [37] Indeed, the biphasal action of drugs on the human and animal organism is an ignored topic in modern allopathic pharmacological treatises. And yet it is a rather pervasive phenomenon which is frequently mentioned in anecdotal accounts of pharmacological (and other) trials. °

The following examples are only a representative selection.

Duke in 1915 reported on experiments to influence the platelet count in rabbits by injecting them with toxins, bacterial emulsions, or chemical poisons in varying doses. "It was possible to reduce the platelet count by using a large dose of any agent which in smaller doses caused a rise in the count, and vice versa. . . . The agents with which it was possible to produce the most rapid and extreme rises in the count, namely, diphtheria toxin and benzol, were also the ones with which the most rapid and extreme falls in the count were produced. . . . The most powerful stimulants are also the most powerful poisons, as a rule." [38]

Perfusion of kitten heart with dilute cobra venom (1971) is seen to have the following effects: a concentration of 1:150,000 stimulates the heartbeat, a concentration of 1:60,000 stimulates it slightly while decreasing the amplitude, one of 1:30,000 causes irregular beats of shorter amplitude, 1:27,000 makes the beat quite irregular and decreases the amplitude, and a concentration of 1:15,000 stops the beat entirely.[39]

Searle in 1920 found that colloidal copper injected intravenously in large doses aggravates boils; injected intramuscularly in smaller doses it causes them to heal.[40]

Wolf in 1940 stated that glandular extracts in small doses

---

° The living organism undoubtedly reacts biphasally to *all* external stimuli, not merely the subclass represented by medicinal drugs and X-rays. Selye notes that the "stress reaction" or "general adaptation syndrome" is itself biphasal: exposure to stress first evokes an "alarm reaction" which is followed by a "stage of resistance." "The manifestations of this second stage were quite different from, and, in many instances the exact opposite of, those which characterized the alarm reaction." The "alarm reaction" is described by Selye as the "primary change, or damage," while the "stage of resistance" is characterized as the "secondary change, or defense" (Hans Selye, *The Stress of Life*, Revised Edition. [New York: McGraw-Hill, 1978], 37, 71).

stimulate an activity while larger doses act to depress that activity.[41]

Seiffert in 1928 reported that many substances used in treating infectious diseases act *in vivo* against microorganisms much more intensely in small doses than in large ones.[42]

Almroth Wright, a pioneer of immunology, pointed out early in this century that there is a great difference between large and small doses of vaccine in the treatment of typhoid. If a very small dose is employed, such as to cause very slight constitutional disturbance, there is a brief "negative" phase of diminished bactericidal power in the patient's blood. Where the dose is larger, the "negative" phase lasts longer; and when a very large dose of vaccine is used, the negative phase is extremely prolonged — perhaps indefinitely.[43] In the same vein, modern medicine accepts the concept of antigenic or immunologic "tolerance" — meaning failure of the immunologic system to respond to a massive dose of an antigen which, in a small dose, will evoke a profound reaction.

Alexander Fleming observed in 1946 that in early work on sulfanilamide complete bacteriostasis was achieved with a small *in vitro* inoculum, while the microbes grew freely if the inoculum was large.[44] Garrod in 1951 observed that the use of chemotherapeutic drugs in concentrations lower than those required to inhibit growth of bacteria can actually stimulate growth of these same bacteria.[45] This suggests that the so-called "superinfections" and emergence of "drug resistant" bacterial strains observed in modern hospital practice may be due, in part, to *stimulation* of such bacteria by the chemo-therapeutic drugs employed so widely.

Eppinger in 1934 observed that four to five minutes after injection with adrenalin the blood pressure is briefly lower than prior to the injection.[46] A 1960 letter to the editor of the AMA *Journal* elicited the response that a subcutaneous injection of 1 cc. of the 1:1000 solution of epinephrine causes vasodilation and decreased cardiac output.[47]

The opposite effects of high and low doses of X-radiation have been reported by several workers. Duke noted this in connection with his work on the platelet count in rabbits.[48] Taylor and Weld (1931) noted that the effect of irradiated ergosterol on calcium metabolism is reversed as the dose is increased from small to very large amounts.[49] Workers in the

Strangeways Laboratory of Cambridge University found that the minimum dose of gamma rays sufficient to affect cellular mitosis at first caused a reduction, but that this reduction was then followed by a compensatory increase.[50] The International Atomic Energy Agency reported in 1963 that the sperm of insects sterilized by low doses of nitrogen mustard had the capacity to fertilize more eggs than normal (yielding sterile eggs).[51] A similar effect was found in the chemical sterilization of male flies with apholate: they turned out to be more sexually aggressive than unsterilized flies and produced more (sterile) eggs.[52]

Wilder himself adduced a series of instances in support of his law.

Novocaine, which in large doses stimulates the central nervous system, nevertheless counteracts the tonic phase of the electroshock convulsion, as do benzadrine and other similar substances.[53] All organs, and especially the nervous system, are, up to a point, more sensitive to stimuli under narcosis, and paradoxical reactions are often encountered; this is true for the respiration of plants under the influence of various narcotics, and even for enzymes.[54] Additional doses of the same narcotic, or addition of another narcotic at a certain point of the narcosis (a certain initial level), reverses the narcotic effect of the previous dose.[55] Tranquilizers often tend to excite the patient rather than calm him.[56] Ataractics have paradoxical effects: thus, chlorpromazine may stop or cause nausea, depress or elevate the temperature, etc.[57] The dose-response effect of amphetamine on locomotor activity in mammals such as the rat takes the form of a U-shaped function: low doses increase locomotor activity, while high doses cause an apparent reduction in behavioral output.[58] Cortisone and ACTH have dual psychotic effects — both manic and depressive.[59] Hypertension has been treated successfully with adrenalin.[60] Under the effect of electroshock or novocaine, capillary fragility — considered as an indication of stress — rises if it was initially low but drops if it was initially elevated.[61] Fear has been shown to raise or depress the number of blood leucocytes as an inverse function of their initial value, i.e., increasing them when they were few in number and decreasing them when they were numerous.[62]

Rinkel commented recently that

A major difficulty . . . of drug and biochemical studies in general is the fact that the same substance administered in different concentrations or for different lengths of time may have different, and even quite opposite, effects. This situation also applies in *in vitro* studies of cells and of isolated enzyme systems and is more complicated when one deals with the intact organism as a whole. Reasonable chemical hypotheses for these quantitative relationships have been advanced, but a clear understanding of drug action is still for the future.[63]

Often the phenomenon of reversal of effect is described as "paradoxical."

Drugs such as dextroamphetamine or methylphenidate are stimulants, arousing the metabolism and increasing alertness. When used to excess, they can cause overstimulation, restlessness, insomnia, agitation, etc. And yet these substances have been found useful in treating hyperkinetic children. The HEW *Report of the Conference on the Use of Stimulant Drugs in the Treatment of Behaviorally Disturbed Young School Children* (1971) noted that "much has been made of the 'paradoxical sedative' effect of stimulants in such children." [64]

A similar instance is the use of coffee in the hyperkinetic child. Schnackenberg found that hyperkinetic children tend to drink coffee more than usual and, when asked why, respond, "It calms me down" or "I can do better in school." [65]

The relationship between iodine and goiter is full of paradoxes. Goiter is well known to be caused by insufficient iodine in the diet. At the same time, administration of iodine salts in excess causes both hyperthyroidism and myxoedema with goiter.[66] A modern authority writes: "A curious and as yet not fully explained antithyroidal effect is produced by large doses of iodides; for example, in man ¼ to ½ g. of potassium iodide a day, or several hundred times the normal daily intake. This effect has been made use of in the treatment of hyperthyroidism." [67]

In 1969 physicians in the Hartford Burn Clinic reported excellent effects from the use of a .5% silver nitrate solution, applied twice a day, in deep third-degree burns. There was absence of pain, control of infection, ease of management, formation of eschars that separated painlessly, and better acceptance of skin grafts. Silver nitrate, of course, is used in large doses to burn off erosions of the cervix, warts, etc., so its use in burn treatment must be considered "paradoxical." The authors warn that a solution stronger than .5% will necrotize and destroy the tissue.[68]

The use of X-rays for treating cancer and tumors could be considered paradoxical (as it was when initially introduced), since such radiation is known to cause tumors and cancers. It is perhaps significant that the first person to make therapeutic use of X-rays for this purpose was Emil Grubbe, a professor of chemistry and a student at the (homoeopathic) Hahnemann Medical College of Chicago. He treated breast cancer and lupus with X-rays in 1896.[69]

Clearly this issue of the opposite effects caused by the same medicine under different circumstances is far from having been exhausted by modern allopathic medicine. Homoeopathy, however, avoids the problem by assuming that the "biphasal" action of drugs is merely an instance of a more general phenomenon — the compensatory reaction developed by the living organism to a morbific stimulus. Homoeopathic medical practice works to strengthen and support this compensatory reaction.

Part of the resistance in conventional medicine to the concept that drugs have a dual action doubtless stems from the assumption that drugs do not act on the body of the patient but rather on the "disease" or, at least, on the microorganism assumed to be the disease cause. Homoeopathy has always maintained that medicines act only on the body of the patient, stimulating a reaction. Even in the case of disease processes associated with microorganisms homoeopathy considers that the medicine stimulates the body's defenses, and these, in turn, act to suppress the microorganisms.

While conventional medicine has generally adhered to the first view above, the alternative — homoeopathic — interpretation of drug action also figures there. Throughout the 1920's and 1930's, for example, a dispute was carried on between those who ascribed the curative effect of mercurial medicines in syphilis to their direct action on the spirochete and those who felt that these medicines stimulated the defensive reaction of the host. Alexander Fleming wrote in 1946, after the dispute had been settled in favor of the latter view: "there were no tests proving that [mercury] ever reached the circulation in concentrations inimical to the spirochete, but from the clinical results we may presume that something happened after a strenuous course of mercury which influenced the disease."[70]

A similar dispute raged at the same time over the action of quinine in malaria. While this medicine was initially considered to act directly against the malaria microorganism (plasmodium), research in the 1920's and 1930's showed that the levels of quinine attained in the blood during treatment (less than 1:24,000) were far too low to kill the plasmodium *in vitro* (1:5000).[71] After much discussion of how this could be so, the subject was eventually abandoned. The *Encyclopedia Britannica* wrote about quinine in 1957:

> The manner of its highly specific action on the malaria parasite was still not clearly understood at mid-20th century. It does not prevent the establishment of the infection after inoculation by the mosquito (prophylaxis), nor does it cause a complete eradication of the parasites (parasitic cure). Its only action is in suppressing the infection, thus allowing time for the development of the processes of immunity.[72]

This last comment seems compatible with the explanation of the action of quinine given by Hahnemann at the beginning of the nineteenth century.

While it is assumed that the antibiotics used so commonly in modern allopathy act directly against the bacteria or other microorganisms, this may be an inadequate explanation. These antibiotics have been shown to have a stimulant effect on the growth and health of farm animals, increasing vitality and viability, and this may account for at least part of the observed beneficial effect of these medicines in the treatment of disease.[73]

# Chapter Five
# The Provings of Homoeopathic Medicines

Having become convinced of the biphasal action of medicines on the human organism, Hahnemann undertook a program of provings. The proving of medicinal substances on healthy persons, to ascertain their curative powers, is the specific homoeopathic contribution to medicine and the methodological basis of homoeopathic practice.

By the end of the nineteenth century records had been compiled of the provings of about 600 substances, and these have been collected in the classic works of Constantine Hering° and Timothy Field Allen.°° The other standard text in homoeopathic practice is James Tyler Kent's *Repertory of the Homoeopathic Materia Medica*°°° which is based in part upon the compilations of Hering and Allen and constitutes an analytic index of these works.

These three massive compendia, published from 70 to 100 years ago, are still the fundamental materials of the homoeopathic school and the indispensable tools of homoeopathic

---

°*The Guiding Symptoms of Our Materia Medica* (Philadelphia: The American Homoeopathic Publishing Society, 1879-1891), Ten Volumes.
°°*Encyclopedia of Pure Materia Medica* (New York and Philadelphia: Boericke and Tafel, 1874-1880), Eleven Volumes.
°°°This work has had numerous editions and reprintings.

43

medical practice. This is naturally surprising to persons unacquainted with homoeopathy, who regard it as a sign of backwardness to use books of such antiquity. However, the reason for the longevity of the homoeopathic classics is not far to seek. They are the records of *symptoms*. While theories of disease etiology, and of the pathological or biochemical involvement of the internal organs and tissues, change from decade to decade with the movement of medical thought, the symptoms manifested by the sick patient are unchanging. Provers today will display precisely the same symptoms as those of the nineteenth century when exposed to the same medicinal substances. Hence the homoeopathic records of provings are as up-to-date today as they were at the time of their first appearance.

But research on the provings did not come to an end with publication of the works of Hering and Allen. Several hundred other substances have been proven since that time, more or less fully, and this information is also available in the homoeopathic publications.

One prominent collection of 20th-century provings is James Stephenson's *Hahnemannian Provings, 1924-1959, A Materia Medica and Repertory* (Bombay, 1963), containing the symptoms of: *Alloxan*, amniotic fluid, *Araneus ixobolus, Aristolochia clematitis, Bellis perennis, Beryllium metallicum, Buthus australis, Butyricum acidum, Cadmium metallicum, Calcarea fluorica, Carcinosin, Cobaltum nitricum, Corticotropin*, cortisone, *Cytisus scoparius*, sarcolactic acid, *Eysenhardtia polystachia (Ortega), Guatteria gaumeria, Hedera helix, Hippuricum acidum, Histaminum hydrochloricum, Ipomea stans. cav., Laburnum anagyroides, Latrodectus mactans, Lophophora Williamsii, Magnesium sulphuricum, Mandragora officinarum, Natrum fluoricum, Ocimum sanctum*, posterior pituitary gland, *Rauwolfia serpentina, Strophanthus sarmentosus*, sulfanilamide, *Taraxacum, Thymol, Viscum album*, and *X-ray*. Stephenson also points out that the homoeopathic provings are by no means complete: for example, only 41 of the inorganic chemical elements have been proven, while more than 50 still remain.[74]

The view has sometimes been expressed that the homoeopathic proving method is not "scientific" in, allegedly, not being subject to control for the observational and repertorial skills of the provers or even their honesty in reporting symptoms or failing to report them. Doubt has been cast on the provings of such supposedly inert substances as silica or others — like sodium chloride (table salt), presumed devoid of therapeutic power.

In its extreme form this argument would hold that twenty or thirty volumes of homoeopathic provings are a fabrication, a figment of the nineteenth-century medico-religious imagination. Indeed, the interpretation of homeopathy given by some of the allopathic medical historians is not far from this.

Fortunately, such allegations are not difficult to disprove.

In the first place, it can hardly be denied that *some* substances, in particular those known as "poisons," do affect the organism in a way which is typical and characteristic of each such "poison." The homoeopathic provings of poisonous substances, of which there are a considerable number, do, in fact, reveal the typical poisoning symptoms, not because the provers are sacrificed for science but because these same poisoning symptoms appear in a milder form during proving with a highly diluted poison. For instance, the proving of the saliva of a rabid dog (*Hydrophobinum*) yields such symptoms as "a large quantity of viscid saliva in mouth, causing me to spit an unusual quantity" and "slight sore throat, difficulty in swallowing liquids" — milder forms of the typical "foaming at the mouth" and hydrophobia of the rabid animal.[75]

On a more mundane level, the proving of strychnine (*Strychnos nux vomica*) gives, *inter alia*, "sensitive to all impressions," "jaws contracted," "spasmodic constriction [of the breathing]," "shallow respiration," "oppressed breathing."[76] And a modern treatise on poisoning gives as symptoms of strychnine poisoning: "feeling of uneasiness and heightened sensibility to external stimuli," "strange feeling in the jaw muscles," "catching of the respiration," etc.[77]

The proving symptoms of *Aconitum napellus* include, *inter alia*, "red, dry, constricted . . . burning throat," "cold sweat . . . cold waves pass through him," "oppressed breathing on least motion," "weak and lax ligaments of all joints," "retention of urine."[78] The above-mentioned treatise on poisoning gives for aconite: "feeling of constriction and

45

burning extending from mouth to stomach," "cold," "anxious oppressive feeling in chest," "cold sweat," "muscular weakness," "no urine." [79]

The provings of *Belladonna* include: "pupils dilated," "throat dry, as if glazed," "difficult deglutition," "hoarse, loss of voice," "ocular illusions," "spasms," "delirium." [80] The treatise on poisons gives: "dilatation of pupils," "dryness of mouth and throat," "difficulty swallowing," "change in voice (hoarseness)," "derangement of vision," "clonic spasms," "in delirium picks at clothes and talks to self." [81]

While the provings of these substances yield hundreds more symptoms, the overall picture is close enough to the ordinary descriptions of poisonings in the medical literature to place beyond any doubt the accuracy of the homoeopathic observations.

But it will then be alleged that poisons are a special case and that non-poisons do not yield such a variety of symptoms. The homoeopathic answer to this is that the distinction between "poisons" and "non-poisons" is arbitrary — not a matter of the essence of the substance but purely one of the quantity ingested. Hahnemann wrote in 1806 that no substance is poisonous when taken in its correct dose. [82] A "poison" is a substance which is harmful to the organism even in small doses; at the same time, such otherwise innocuous substances as table salt can be "poisonous" if consumed in large amounts. The more powerful the effect of a substance on the living organism, the smaller the toxic, and, *a fortiori*, the therapeutic, dose.

Thus the "poison," the "medicine," and the supposedly "inert substance" lie along a spectrum — their effect on the organism being determined by their dose and mode of preparation, in perfect harmony with the Arndt-Schulz and Koetschau rules.

Indeed, the supposedly "inert" substances used in homoeopathy, have occasionally been the object of ridicule. Everyone knows, for instance, that ingested grains of sand will pass through the body without producing a discernible effect. However, when the sand is ground up very fine, it can have an effect. L. U. Gardner reported in 1937 that the inhalation of fine particles of silica by guinea pigs, or their injection in colloidal form, can cause serious and even lethal pathology.

"Silica can cause every type of cellular response found in tuberculosis."[°][83] Miners breathing silica dust are known, furthermore, to develop scleroderma (hardening of the skin), polyarthritis, and involvement of the lungs, heart, and kidneys.[84]

In an experiment, to be described below, on 200 guinea pigs, systematic administration of table salt in a high dilution produced marked pathology in the test group, lowered weight, and higher morbidity and mortality.[85]

A further objection to the provings might be that they contain masses of extraneous data attributable solely to the prover's imagination or to his particular idiosyncrasy.

This is a serious theoretical issue. When a prover takes a medicinal substance for a period of time, are all of his subsequent symptoms, feelings, and sensations to be ascribed to the effect of this substance? Or can some be ignored on the ground that they relate to the prover's idiosyncrasy or imagination?

Hahnemann himself laid down the condition that the prover should be healthy, not suffering from any illness. Then whatever symptoms he manifested after ingesting the substance (until the end of the period during which it was known to be active) were to be regarded as the effects of the substance.

In support of Hahnemann it must be admitted that to distinguish between the symptoms caused by such a substance and those not caused by it, but appearing after ingestion of the substance, is impossible. To state that certain symptoms are the fruit of the prover's imagination is no answer, since the substance might be working through his imagination. To state that it is the effect of idiosyncrasy is also no answer, since who of us does not have some physical or mental idiosyncrasy? Medicines are continually being used to treat persons with idiosyncrasies, and in homoeopathy the symptoms of the individual's idiosyncrasy are precisely the most useful ones.

Despite this theoretical argument, however, the homoeo-

° *Silica* in homoeopathy is known to have such an affinity for the pulmonary tuberculous process that the prescriber is expressly warned of this danger: "In phthisis [*Silica*] must be used with care, for here it may cause the absorption of scar-tissue, liberate the disease, walled in, to new activities" (William Boericke, *Materia Medica with Repertory*, Ninth Edition, 590).

pathic physicians engaged in provings have attempted to exert some control over the symptoms reported. The problem of ensuring accuracy in the reporting of symptoms was commented on as follows by Hering:

> We certainly cannot do anything except to find some observations more, and others less, probable, and, of course, confirmation increases the probability until a higher law decides. . . . It is fifty years now since I joined the Homoeopathic School, and I have never met a single prover who "believed" the symptoms he obtained and who did not seek confirmations. We not only repeated experiments again and again, but we were anxious to have other provers, and if their results were published, we always compared anxiously those of others with our own. . . . What we had repeatedly found confirmed by cures, day after day, week after week, and year after year, is what we took as our basis, as a true gain in the new science; these were what we called the characteristics of the drug.[86]

If homoeopathy is not to be shifted from its reliance on symptoms to some other basis (in which case it would cease being homoeopathy), the method of registering symptoms set forth by Hahnemann and Hering and practiced for more than 175 years will have to be left alone. It cannot be criticized as inherently false or inaccurate even though, like any technique for gathering and recording data, it is sometimes difficult to apply. The ultimate test of the proving method is therapeutic practice, and homoeopathy has found this practice to be more than satisfactory.

If further evidence is needed of the validity of the homoeopathic provings, it may be noted that some of the homoeopathic substances have been proved a second time under controlled conditions, with the provers not knowing which substance they were ingesting. The results have only confirmed the original data.

The best example is the reproving of *Belladonna* done in the beginning of the twentieth century under the auspices of the American Homoeopathic Ophthalmological, Otological, and Laryngological Society.[87]

For this reproving a central director was appointed (Howard Bellows, professor of otology at the Boston University School of Medicine), with regional and associate directors in ten major cities. Fifty provers were recruited, and in each of these cities they were examined during the course of the proving by homoeopathic specialists. Neither the provers themselves nor these specialists knew that the reproving was of *Belladonna*. The provers recorded their symptoms from day to day and went periodically to discuss them with the specialists. They also discussed them with the regional director (who knew that the drug being proved was *Belladonna*).

Thus the reproving of *Belladonna* was partly "blind" in the sense that the provers themselves and the special examiners (who did most of the verification of symptoms) did not know what the substance was. Furthermore, it was controlled in that the provers were initially given placebo and only after a few days were transferred to *Belladonna*. The director, Howard Bellows, stated: "that the prover should not know when he is taking a drug and when a blank, I believe all will agree, is most reasonable and is, indeed, an absolute necessity for scientific accuracy." [88]

The result was a book of 665 pages, of which 121 contain a condensed list of the symptoms recorded. The pattern is identical with the symptomatology of *Belladonna* given in the nineteenth-century texts. This would appear to indicate that the earlier provers did their work well.

Other substances have been reproved in more recent decades, although in a less comprehensive fashion. Since 1945 the *Journal of the American Institute of Homoeopathy* has presented reprovings of Peruvian Bark,[89] *Thuja*,[90] *Taraxacum officinale*,[91] *Cinchona officinalis*,[92] *Cactus Grandiflorus*,[93] and others.[94] Again, the patterns obtained in the reprovings have been similar or identical to those obtained in the nineteenth century.

# Chapter Six

# The Organism's Ultrasensitivity
# to the Similar Medicine

Another of the fruitful concepts introduced into medicine by Hahnemann was that the patient is hypersensitive to the similar medicine. In this way he explained the effectiveness of his very small doses.

And since the similar remedy stimulates the patient's existing symptom-pattern, its administration is usually followed by a momentary aggravation of the symptoms.

Both of these concepts are accepted in conventional medicine.

Hypersensitivity was rediscovered in 1891 by Robert Koch who noted that tuberculin could be injected in considerable quantities into normal animals, while tuberculous animals reacted very violently, even to small doses, some dying within a few hours.[95] Hypersensitivity was initially associated with infectious disease, but Portier and Richet in 1902 showed that hypersensitivity (anaphylaxis) could be produced by repeated injections of albumin. The hypersensitive state then came to be understood as representing the body's reaction to any external insult, not only to highly toxic or infectious substances. It is found in various diseases.[96] The assumption that only a protein is capable of inducing hypersensitivity broke down with Landsteiner's discovery that non-antigenic substances can unite chemically with a protein "carrier" and thus become antigens. And today the problem of drug hyper-sensitivity raises the possibility that hypersensitization arises in a variety of ways, not only through introduction of a protein into the organism.[97]

The hyper-reactivity, or symptom-aggravation, of the hypersensitive organism when exposed to the "similar" remedy is also discussed in the allopathic medical literature. Crowe, who treated rheumatic diseases with vaccines made from the bacteria associated with the disease, noted the extreme sensitivity of his patients — compelling him to reduce his doses to levels many times lower than those earlier employed.[98] Walbum, who in the 1920's developed a technique of treating infectious diseases with injections of colloidal metals, found an inverse relationship between the curative effect of the injection and the degree of aggravation; he reduced his doses to the level which minimized the aggravation and found that this yielded optimum therapeutic results.[99] The well-known Jarisch-Herxheimer reaction in the treatment of syphilis — fever, headache, malaise, and sweating commencing 2-12 hours after the initiation of treatment and lasting one day — is doubtless an instance of therapeutic aggravation of symptoms. It was noted when syphilis was treated with arsphenamine, and it is still noted today with treatment by penicillin.[100]

The concepts of sensitivity and therapeutic aggravation of symptoms in the presence of the "similar" medicine are quite common in immunology and allergology. Crowe in 1931 observed that the vaccine treatment of chronic rheumatic disease often gives rise to an initial aggravation, which is to be considered a positive phenomenon.[101] Zinsser stated the same in his text on immunology.[102] Writers on the treatment of allergy stress that the desensitizing dose is the one just below the dose which causes an aggravation (i.e., Koetschau's A curve where the "primary symptoms" are not apparent, and only the "secondary symptoms" are seen).[103]

# Chapter Seven
# The Infinitesimal Dose

Homoeopathy is most closely associated in the public mind with the supposedly "illogical" principle that the power of a medicine increases with dilution, and with the corollary of this principle: that the greatest power is to be found in the small or infinitesimal dose.

These have been major points of criticism by non-homoeopathic physicians. And, indeed, both of these principles have been sources of amazement to the homoeopathic physicians themselves (who are medically well-informed and fully aware of the scientific issues involved).

### (a) Evidence for the Infinitesimal Dose

Clinical experience with these small doses has always stimulated the scientific curiosity of homoeopathic investigators, and, since the early decades of the twentieth century, they have sponsored a variety of physical, chemical, botanical, and biological experiments in an effort to demonstrate the existence of some medicinal power in them.

It should be made clear at the outset that the use of the small, or ultramolecular, dose is not an integral part of homoeopathic doctrine. The accepted rule is that the physician should employ the "minimum dose" capable of eliciting the desired response, and Hahnemann himself employed tinctures as well as medicines at all stages of dilution.

The "infinitesimal" dose was only an empirical discovery by Hahnemann. When he administered medicines according to the law of similars, he found that the patients reacted very violently (their "primary symptoms," Koetschau's B and C curves), and he reduced his doses in order to moderate the patient's reaction.

Allopathic medicine should not be amazed at the homoeopathic small doses, since the power of minute quantities is recognized today outside homoeopathy as well as inside it. A milligram of acetylcholine dissolved in 500,000 gallons of blood can lower the blood pressure of a cat; even smaller amounts will affect the beat of a frog's heart.[104] Florey reported in 1943 that pure penicillin will inhibit the development of sensitive microorganisms *in vitro* at dilutions of 1:50,000,000 to 1:100,000,000; morphological effects on streptococci were seen at dilutions of 1:250,000,000.[105] Fleming noted that diluting penicillin 80,000,000 times was like taking one drop of water and dividing it among "over 6000 whisky bottles."[106] Zinsser found that sensitization could be achieved with 1/1,000,000 of a cc. of horse serum, and with even smaller quantities of egg albumin.[107] The human body manufactures 50-100 millionths of a gram of thyroid hormone per day, and the concentration of free thyroid hormone in the normal blood is one part per 10,000 million parts of blood plasma.[108]

Hahnemann was a contemporary of Amadeo Avogadro who discovered that the number of molecules in one mole of any substance is $6.0253 \times 10^{23}$. Once the existence of this Avogadro Constant had penetrated the medical consciousness, orthodox physicians turned from criticism of the homoeopathic small doses to criticism of the ultramolecular dose, since it became clear that medicines diluted beyond $10^{-23}$ — i.e., the 12C or 24X dilutions — fell outside the range within which it could be expected that a single molecule of the original medicinal substance remained in the dilution.

In the following pages we will present some of the experiments done to demonstrate the existence of a force (of undefined nature) in the homoeopathic small doses, including those diluted beyond the Avogadro Limit.

53

## (i) Biochemical Investigations

The most striking experiment conducted under homoeopathic auspices to demonstrate the power of the "high dilutions" was that of William Boyd in Edinburgh, published in 1954.[109]

In the early 1930's V. M. Persson in Leningrad had investigated microdilutions (up to 120X) of mercuric chloride for their effect on the fermentation of starch by salivary amylase and on the lysis of fibrin by pepsin and trypsin, obtaining significant results in controlled studies.[110] In 1933 he repeated the experiments and published new confirmatory observations.[111]

The purpose of Boyd's experiments was to confirm Persson's results. He repeated the experiments with fanatical attention to procedural detail and after making every conceivable effort to eliminate observer bias (the description of this experiment, which is rather simple in principle, takes 53 pages in the *Journal of the American Institute of Homeopathy*).

The microdilutions used were mercuric chloride 61X ($10^{-61}$) which, by present physical theory, should contain no molecules of the original mercuric chloride but only the distilled water used as diluent.

The experiment sought to establish whether addition of a small quantity of mercuric chloride microdilution affected the speed of hydrolysis of starch with diastase. Control flasks containing starch, diastase, and distilled water were compared with flasks containing these plus the mercuric chloride microdose. The rates of hydrolysis were studied colorimetrically with an absorptiometer, and since the results showed biological scatter, the frequencies of the differences were analyzed statistically.

The experiment showed that addition of mercuric chloride 61X accelerated the rate of hydrolysis.

Boyd conducted more than 500 comparisons, in several series from 1946 to 1952. Analysis was done by independent statisticians who reported that they showed significance (P less than .001). One wrote: "significant difference is shown from the controls by every set of the series. The probabilities are very strong indeed. This means that there is certainly a difference between your solutions and the controls."

The minutest precautions were taken to avoid error and to

ensure that the experimental conditions remained unchanged.

The laboratory temperature was thermostatically controlled. The air was filtered at input and extracted by a fan.

The temperature of incubation of the starch mixture was controlled to within 0.005 degrees centigrade.

The glass bottles and jars used were systematically interchanged between test and control groups to exclude the possibility of absorption of mercuric chloride as a cause of the observed differences between test and control series.

A very complex procedure was utilized for boiling the glassware, involving multiple washing in distilled water and baking for 2½ hours in an oven at 150° centigrade.

A single-blind procedure was employed in that the technician dosing the starch solution with either mercuric chloride or distilled water did not know which bottle contained which until after completion of the series.

It was necessary to train a technician for 18 months before she was able to perform all the procedures with the requisite accuracy.

The outcome of this experiment was reported in extenso in *The Pharmaceutical Journal* (September 11, 1954) which quoted the president of the (London) Faculty of Homeopathy to the effect that this "would prove to be one of the greatest medical advances recorded." Reports appeared also in the British newspapers.[112]

Experiments similar to Boyd's, and controlled in the same way, have been performed by homoeopathic physicians in France, although with "lower" dilutions, Lacharme *et al.* in 1965 showed that a 3C dilution of *Physostigma venenosa* accelerates the acetyl-cholinesterase reaction.[113] Boiron and Marin in the same year showed that low decimal dilutions of sodium fluoride affect the hydrolysis of saccharose by invertase.[114]

## (ii) Botanical Investigations

A number of well-controlled botanical experiments have been performed by homoeopathic investigators, the reason perhaps being (as stated by one French physician) — "is there anyone who will claim a placebo effect on plants?"[115]

Kolisko, in 1923, was a pioneer in this field, soaking wheat seeds and others in microdilutions (up to $10^{-30}$) of such substances as iron sulfate, antimony trioxide, and a double-salt of copper. She found that growth was promoted by the lower dilutions, then inhibited with higher dilutions, and then again stimulated at even higher dilutions. Both measurement and weighing of the shoots gave the same result. Her work continued for decades, and a full report of all her experiments was published in 1959.[116]

She was followed in this by Wilhelm Pelikan and Georg Unger who published similar results in 1965.[117] One of their experiments investigated the effects of microdoses of silver nitrate on the growth of wheat seeds. It tested the effect of 12 different microdoses of silver nitrate (8X to 19X), plus one control, on the germination and sprouting of the seeds; the series was repeated 240 times, and statistical analysis of the results showed the effect of the different potencies. The length of shoots increased from 8X to 11X, then dropped at 12X, rose again through 13X and 14X, dropped at 16X, rose at 17X and 18X, and dropped at 19X. Thus the effects of progressively "higher" potencies took the form of a sinusoidal curve.[118]

Joseph Roy in 1932 made microdilutions of barley stems, then soaked barley seeds in these dilutions before planting them. He found that the 3C, 6C, 9C, 12C, and 18C microdilutions each gave a different weight of barley shoots as compared with the controls.[119]

Boiron and Zervudacki soaked wheat seeds in water and allowed them to germinate for three days; then they cut off the shoots and soaked them in either distilled water (the controls) or various microdilutions of sodium arsenate ($AsO_4Na_2H$). They found that the subsequent emission of oxygen by the shoots was affected by the microdilution used: 3X, 4X, and 5X were strongly inhibiting, 10X, 12X, and 14X had no particular effect, while 16X and 18X were very stimulating.[120] These experiments were duplicated by Boiron and Marin.[121]

Netien performed a different set of experiments, using as test material the peas from plants raised in soil heavily impregnated with copper sulfate. After determining that the germination potential (i.e., the proportion of peas germinating in a given period of time) was the same for these as for peas raised under normal conditions (used as controls), he soaked the controls and half the test peas in bidistilled water for 24 hours, while the rest of the test peas were soaked for the same period of time in various microdilutions (5X, 7X, 9X, and 15X) of copper sulfate. After three days the test peas had germinated slightly further than the control peas, but no difference could be detected between the test peas soaked in water and those soaked in the various microdilutions. Then the batches of shoots were soaked in microdilutions corresponding to the microdilutions in which the peas themselves had initially been soaked. The subsequent development of the sprouts then varied considerably from the controls, with all of the batches of test material showing much greater development of roots and branches. The author's photographs are quite convincing.[122] This experiment was duplicated by Boiron and Gravioux with wheat seeds soaked in arsenical solutions.[123]

Netien, Boiron, and Marin performed a similar experiment with pea plants impregnated with copper sulfate, showing that addition of copper sulfate microdilutions to the growth medium intensified the excretion of copper by the plants.[124]

In the United States Wannamaker conducted experiments over a period of years to test the effect of sulphur microdilutions on the growth of onion plants. She planted seedlings obtained from a commercial grower in large trays, 96 seedlings per tray, and added 12X, 24X, 30C, 60X, and 20M sulphur microdilutions to the trays. Trays were also set aside as controls. The microdilutions were found to affect, in a significant way, the weight and dimensions of the onion bulbs and seedlings, and also their calcium, magnesium, potassium, and sodium content.[125]

Wannamaker has performed similar experiments measuring the effect of boron microdilutions on onion growth; she concludes that the weight and length of the plants are affected, as well as their boron and sulphur content.[126]

### (iii) Bacteriological Investigations

H. Junker, in 1927, investigated the effect of various microdilutions on paramecia cultures. He added microdilutions, up to $10^{-27}$, of cocaine sulfate, atropin sulfate, caffeine, orange juice, lemon juice, a sodium salt, potassium oleate, octyl alcohol, oleic acid, hydrochloric acid, acetic acid, uric acid, magnesium sulfate, copper sulfate, nonylic acid, sodium desoxycholate and others, and found that differences —

measured in terms of the daily changes in growth of each paramecia culture in function of the degree of dilution of the substance added — took the typical sinusoidal form found by other investigators.[127]

Patterson and Boyd in 1941 reported alteration of the Schick test from positive to negative following peroral administration of alum precipitated toxoid 30C or *Diphtherinum* 201C (made from diphtheria bacillus).[128]

### (iv) Zoological Investigations

Krawkow in 1923 was apparently the first to use homoeopathic microdilutions in experiments on animals, investigating their effect on the blood supply of the isolated rabbit ear. He connected the ear arteries through rubber tubes to a bottle containing Ringer's lactate and compared the flow of the lactate with and without addition of various microdilutions. Bichloride of mercury 24X gave a 30% reduction in blood flow in one trial and a 22% increase in another. Histamine 30X gave a 23% reduction in blood flow. Strychnine nitrate gave a 7% increase etc. Krawkow, moreover, noted a biphasal effect: many poisons in relatively strong concentrations widened the capillaries, while in weaker ones they narrowed them, and vice-versa. Typical vasoconstrictors such as adrenalin and histamine relaxed the capillaries in small doses; chloroform, ether, and other narcotics which widen the capillaries in large doses narrowed them in small doses.[129]

Stearns in New York (1925) added arsenic trioxide *(Arsenicum album)*, mercuric nitrate, and triturated tumor material, in microdilutions of from 6X to 400X, to cultures of fruit flies (Drosophila melanogaster) of a strain in which approximately half of all males died of an inherited tumor. Addition of microdilution caused a reduction in the male death rate from inherited tumor, the difference being approximately four times greater than in the controls. Of 218 separate larva cultures 22 were used as controls.[130]

In that same year Stearns reported two series of experiments on a total of 212 guinea pigs, of which 147 were used in the trial and 65 retained as controls. The animals were grouped in pens containing three males and 12 females and allowed to live the normal guinea-pig life except that the test animals were given daily doses of sodium chloride 30X, 200X, 400X, 600X, 800X, 1000X, 1200X, and 1400X in distilled water, while the controls received only the distilled water. The trial was run two years in succession, its duration being about six months in each case. Stearns noted that the test animals: 1) lost appetite, 2) lost weight, 3) were less active than the controls, 4) sat in odd positions as though losing the strength of their legs, 5) had dull and shaggy coats, 6) had dull and watery eyes, 7) had a lower reproduction rate and higher death rate than the controls, and 8) gave birth to young weighing less than those of the controls.[131]

Koenig in 1927 raised tadpole embryos in water to which microdilutions of lead nitrate or silver nitrate had been added and measured how many died in a given period. He found differing responses to differing degrees of dilution. Lead nitrate gave low death rates at the 1X, 2X, 3X, 13-16X, 21X, 24X, and 26-29X. High death rates were registered at 5X, 8X, 20X, 23X, 25X, and 30X. Thus the sinusoidal curve of effects was discovered here also. In addition, the 5X dilution of lead nitrate and the 26X dilution of silver nitrate caused early metamorphosis of all tadpoles.[132]

In 1929 Vondracek repeated Koenig's experiment, using Prague city water and gold chloride microdilutions (from 4X to 24X). Mortality was measured throughout the whole period of the trial — 48 days, being calculated as the number of tadpoles dying multiplied by the day of the experiment. Five control glasses were used, and mortality was both higher and lower among the test animals than in the controls. The curve of mortality was sinusoidal.[133]

In 1951 Jarricot reported success in experiments altering neuromuscular excitability of isolated frog and turtle heart through perfusion with 18C to 118C dilutions of *Iberis Amara* and the 60X dilution of veratrine sulfate.[134]

In 1954 Boyd reported on *Strophanthus sarmentosus* experiments in frogs, using electronic circuitry to register the heart rate and its response to direct application (at the auriculo-ventricular junction) of a 32C microdilution of *Strophanthus*. Controls received the same injections, but of distilled water only. Out of the 71 frogs, used first as controls and then as test subjects, 2 reacted to the distilled water (2.8%), while 35 reacted to the *Strophanthus* (49.2%).[135]

Bagros and Boiron communicated in 1955 their experiments with 30C microdilutions of ovarian follicular fluid (*Folliculine*) to counteract the effects of large doses of estradiol. The test was performed on about 2000 female rats, divided into test and control groups. All the rats were injected with estradiol, and those in the test group were then injected with microdilutions of *Folliculine*. The authors found that the microdoses of *Folliculine* had an effect on the rats, and that this effect was antagonistic to the effect of estradiol in ponderal doses.[136]

In these same years Lapp, Wurmser, and Ney investigated the effect of infinitesimal doses of poisons on the body's elimination of these same poisons in ponderal doses. They injected guinea pigs with ponderal but sub-lethal doses of arsenic or bismuth and then administered 4C, 5C, or 7C microdoses of arsenic or bismuth; the effect was greatly to increase the quantities of urinated arsenic or bismuth.[137]

In 1961 Mouriquand *et al.* investigated the effect of 7C doses of sodium arsenate on normalization of the vestibular chronologic index in pigeons injected previously with a sub-lethal dose of arsenic. Arsenic microdoses accelerated normalization of vestibular chronaxie while simultaneously increasing the arsenic content of the stools.[138]

In 1964 two non-homoeopaths working in the Pasteur Institute discovered a similar phenomenon: in mice made tolerant to an endotoxin they were able to bring about elimination of the endotoxin by injecting 1/10,000 of a microgram of the endotoxin.[139]

In 1966 Cier and Boiron reported on the prophylactic effect of injections of a 9C dilution of alloxan against the induction of alloxan diabetes. In mice and rabbits preliminary injection of alloxan 9C totally inhibited the hyperglycemic response to a 40 mg/kg injection of alloxan. This same injection moderated the diabetogenic response to a 60 mg/kg alloxan injection, and it was successfully employed in the treatment of alloxan-induced diabetes.[140]

In another publication these authors presented photographs of the Beta-cells in the islets of Langerhans of the test animals.[141]

They reported also on the prophylactic effect of 7C intraperitoneal injections of horse serum against the Arthus phenomenon in rabbits repeatedly injected with horse serum. With ten rabbits in the test sample and ten in the control group, after 7 injections all the controls manifested the Arthus reaction, and only 6 of the test animals. In the same way they succeeded in modifying the Shwartzman reaction by a 7C endotoxin dilution.[142]

Julian and Launey were able to inhibit and modify the effects of a physiologic dose of reserpine (in mice) by preliminary 7C and 9C injections of *Rauwolfia serpentina*. The same experiment was performed successfully with *Cicuta virosa*.[143]

Lallouette and Boyer reported in 1967 on the inhibiting effect of calcium sulphide microdilutions on inflammation and edema provoked by injections of staphylococcal toxin. Other researchers demonstrated the prophylactic effect of endotoxin microdoses (in guinea pigs) against response to histamine aerosols.[144]

J. and M. Tetau reported in 1969 on modifying *Thuja* intoxication in rats by a 9C *Thuja* injection. The rats were first taught a conditioned reflex; then they were injected with *Thuja* to intoxication (shown by loss of the reflex); the test group was then injected with *Thuja* 9C and returned to normalcy (as shown by restoration of the conditioned reflex) more rapidly than the controls.[145]

I. A. Boyd reported in 1968 on the action of a microdilution ($10^{-19}$g/ml) of acetylcholine on the frog heart in a controlled study; he concluded that "certain substances are capable of affecting biological tissues in dilutions which cover a large part of the homeopathic low potency range." Furthermore, that "small amounts of substances may have stimulatory action in the human body when larger amounts have the opposite effect, and that this stimulatory effect may be most marked in diseased or failing tissue."[146]

In 1976 Van Mansvelt and Amons reported on the effect of mercuric chloride, at dilutions as low as $0.9 \times 10^{-25}$, on the proliferation of a mouse lymphoblastic cell strain; growth inhibition was detected down to a level of $0.9 \times 10^{-17}$ but the curve, instead of being flat as expected, had peaks of toxicity at $10^{-5}$, $10^{-6}$, $10^{-16}$, and $10^{-17}$. The authors do not try to explain the findings but call their results a "substantial indication towards some as yet unconceived phenomenon which needs further study."[147] °

### (v) Investigations Using the Techniques of Physics

Wurmser and Loch in 1948 investigated the effect of micro-dilutions on the wave-length and intensity of light from a fixed source. They filtered the light to permit passage of wavelengths from 3800 to 4200 A; this was passed through a receptacle filled with solution, changes being registered by a photoelectric cell. They found measurable changes for quinine sulfate, *Taraxacum dens leonis*, and *Aesculus hippocastanum* at dilutions from 24X to 30X.[148]

In the early 1950's Gay and Boiron found that the dielectric index of distilled water was altered by adding to it a small amount of sodium chloride 27C; by dielectric testing they were able to select the bottle with the sodium chloride microdose out of 99 other bottles containing only distilled water.[149]

Stephenson and Brucato in 1966 repeated Gay's work, measuring changes in the dielectric constant of water to which had been added mercuric chloride in various microdilutions (from 1X to 33X). They found that the dielectric constant was altered from the control for all dilutions up through 33X. The dielectric constant for the control varied between 6.05 and 5.60, with an average at 5.83, while the highest peak attained for any of the microdilutions was 4.40, and the peak for the 33X microdilution was 3.70.[150]

In 1963 Boericke and Smith used nuclear magnetic resonance techniques to investigate the differences among: 1) ordinary 87% hydroalcohol, 2) a 12X dilution of sulphur prepared with succussion at each stage of dilution, and 3) a 12X dilution of sulphur prepared without succussion. They were able to distinguish 2) from 1) and 3) and concluded that

---

° Anyone familiar with this extensive series of homoeopathic animal trials will be startled to read, under the entry "Homoeopathy" in the recently published *Stein and Day International Medical Encyclopedia:* "Although many eminent physicians have given their approval to homoeopathy, it is remarkable that this theory, which could be quite easily put to the test in animal experiments, has never in fact been so tested, and one can only conclude that its practitioners are aware of the fallacies involved."

Homoeopathy since its origin has had to bear the burden of much uninformed criticism similar to the above.

"some form of energy is imparted by succussion to a homoeopathic drug, resulting in a slight change of the alcohol in these dilutions. There is a structural change in the solvent as the potency is made from the tincture to a higher dilution when the solvent is 87% alcohol."[151]

If this preliminary conclusion is correct, it provides an explanation for the observed clinical effect of the homoeopathic ultramolecular dilutions: the "power" of the medicine resides in the solvent phase, not in the solute.

More nuclear magnetic resonance work has been done recently by Young at the Hahnemann Hospital in Philadelphia. Using a 60 Mhz Perkin-Elmer R-12 nuclear magnetic resonance spectrometer he observed changes in alcohol-water solutions as a result of serial dilution and succussion. Dilutions of sulphur, from 5X to 30X, with succussion at each stage, showed measurable changes in the spectra at each stage of dilution and succussion, and the changes followed the sinusoidal curve which seems to be typical in these investigations. The same sinusoidal curve was not detected in Young's investigations of: 1) a series of dilutions of 87% alcohol without any solute added and with rotation at each stage instead of succussion; 2) a series of dilutions of 87% alcohol without any solute and without succussion or rotation at each stage; 3) a series of dilutions of 87% alcohol without any solute added and with succussion at each stage; 4) a series of dilutions of sulphur with rotation at each stage; or 5) a series of sulphur dilutions with neither rotation nor succussion.[152]

### (vi) Theoretical Explanations of the Ultramolecular Dilutions

Several articles outlining a physical theory of the action of the ultramolecular dilutions have been published by Stephenson and Barnard. They suggest that the water phase in the 87% hydroalcohol solution takes on a specific polymeric form reflecting the configuration of the molecules of the solute.

These succussed high dilutions represent stereospecific isotactic polymers imprinted in the solvent by the solute, with self-replicating qualities in the absence of the initial solute. Thus, as in cytoplasmic molecular chemistry, the information content of the solute may reproduce itself separate from its chemical action. As this process may also occur in cellular fluids, it provides an hypothesis for explaining the clinical action of succussed high dilutions, almost on an antigen-antibody basis. [153]

Thus Hahnemann found a "means of separating the structural content of a chemical from its associated chemical mass." [154]

Van Mansvelt and Amons, whose work is mentioned above, also suggest that modifications in the structure of the water used for the serial dilutions of mercuric chloride may permit information to be passed from one dilution to the next. [155]

While this theory of the medicinal action of high potencies is still in the form of a hypothesis, it seems to resemble Bridgman's work on the barometric pressure specificity of ice crystallization patterns in water. [156] He found that water crystallizes in a particular pattern for each barometric pressure, and this pattern reproduces itself when the ice is melted and then refrozen at a lower pressure. The homoeopathic high dilutions thus seem to form part of the area of research dealing with the effect of physical field phenomena on solvents.

### (b) Homoeopathy's Rejection of the Monotonicity Rule

The "monotonicity rule" may be defined as meaning that an increased dose of medicine gives an increased effect while a lower dose gives a lesser effect. This has always been rejected by homoeopathy which holds that: 1) in general, effect is increased by diluting and succussing the substance according to the accepted homoeopathic principles, but 2) more specifically, this increased effect is not a straight-line function of the successive stages of dilution but is sinusoidal (see the discussion on pp. 56-59 above).

Homoeopaths have attempted to explain this phenomenon in terms of the greater fineness of the active medicinal substance in the "higher" potencies — due to their greater degree of trituration. Greater fineness means larger surface area, consequently a larger area of contact between the medicine and the organism of the person ingesting it. But this explanation is inadequate in view of the nuclear magnetic resonance studies discussed above indicating that *succussion* of the medicine at each stage of dilution is an essential step in preparing the homoeopathic medicines and that the water phase of the hydroalcohol is the bearer of the energy of homoeopathic high dilutions.[157]*

Whether or not the homoeopaths have provided a satisfactory explanation for the heightened power of their infinitesimal doses, it is still true that many objections to this homoeopathic principle are based on the unproven assumption that larger doses of medicines always provoke a more powerful response than smaller doses.

In a 1978 article S. H. Kon described this assumption of monotonicity as a rule "of unknown origin, invoked only implicitly, and . . . nameless, unverbalized and unproven for chronic dose-response curves."[158] It is "unproven and unreasonable" in chronic low-toxicity studies. Citing 71 references, Kon concluded that "non-monotonic stimulus-response relationships are common in nature and well explored," that "chronic toxicities of food additives have often been underestimated by those who disregard the experimental data that do not conform to the monotonicity rule," and that "mechanisms of long-term low-level toxicities are unknown."

Of particular interest to homoeopaths is Kon's observation that well-documented effects of low-level exposure have on occasion been simply disregarded by investigators when they did not fit the assumption of monotonicity. He cites the following passages from representative studies:

> tumors . . . occurred only in rats given low doses [of propylene glycol] and thus showed no dose-relationship in their incidence.
>
> Focal hyperplasia . . . occurred with a frequency which was not correlated to increasing doses [of EDTA]. Thus, it may be concluded that these changes were not causally related to test dosage.
>
> Although mortality was highest in the 1% low-dose group

*The homoeopaths attribute enhancement of the medicine's power by succussion to the physical transfer of energy to the medicine. Oddly enough, some support for this idea was provided by an experiment in England comparing two influenza vaccines — one using an ordinary saline solution as its base and the other using an emulsion. The emulsified vaccine acted more powerfully and over a longer period than the saline preparation and with fewer general or local reactions. Although no explanation for this was offered, the formation of an emulsion requires an input of physical energy (see F. Himmelweit, "Serological Responses and Clinical Reactions to Influenza Virus Vaccines," *British Medical Journal*, December, 1960 [ii] 1690-1694).

(all animals dying by the end of the test), no correlation existed between dose-level and mortality. Survival was therefore considered to be unaffected by the intake of coloring [C.I. Food Red No. 5].

Homoeopaths have frequently complained that their results are not accepted by allopathic physicians because they contradict such implicit assumptions as the monotonicity rule. Thus it is a consolation to know that allopathic investigators sometimes reject their own results for the same reason.

While Kon expressly limits his conclusions to long-term chronic exposure, this whole area is unexplored, and his analysis casts doubt on the monotonicity assumption in respect of other dose-response relationships.

# Chapter Eight
# The Single Remedy

Hahnemann advocated the single remedy on practical and theoretical grounds. He thought that the use of medical mixtures led to over-drugging of the patient, but, more specifically, he realized the impossibility of predicting the synergistic effect of several drugs administered simultaneously.

The homoeopathic provings, of course, are all of single substances and chemical compounds (considered as single substances) — never of medicinal mixtures.

This principle has not been adopted by allopathy. Although a voice here and there is raised in opposition to the use of polypharmacal mixtures, e.g.

Nothing could promote more greatly confusion and ineffectiveness of drug therapy than to fix several function-modifiers together. If the dose of the mixture is increased so that function-modifier A produces a maximum therapeutic effect, function-modifier B may already be in highly toxic dosage. Drug A may be rapidly excreted, drug B may be retained in the body ... Physicians who take any drug therapy seriously no longer employ prescriptions in which important function-modifiers are compounded.[159]

More typical is the following:

It is the responsibility of the physician to elicit a good drug history from his patient so that he is aware of what other drugs the patient is receiving and can draw a rational plan as to what medications may be prescribed when they are indicated . . . Because of specialization, many different physicians may see the same patient for several ailments.[160]

# Chapter Nine

# Orthodox Medicine's Use
# of the Law of Similars

The principle of similars is broadly applied in allopathic medicine, being regarded as one of the bases of therapeutics. The whole development of immunology and serum therapy is founded on this principle, as is the specialty of allergology. There are also a number of drugs in common allopathic use whose efficacy is due to the fact that they are employed (unconsciously in most cases) according to the principle of similars.

### (a) Immunology and Serum Therapy

This subject is too extensive, as well as too familiar to the physician, to be developed here, and we may limit ourselves to quoting Emil von Behring, one of the founders of this discipline in the late nineteenth and early twentieth centuries. As the following indicates, he was aware of its close doctrinal relationship to homoeopathy:

In spite of all scientific speculations and experiments concerning smallpox vaccination, Jenner's discovery remained an erratic boulder in medicine until biochemically thinking Pasteur, devoid of all classroom knowledge, traced the origin of this therapeutic boulder to a principle which cannot be better characterized than by Hahnemann's word, "homoeopathic."

Indeed, what else causes the epidemiological immunity in sheep vaccinated against anthrax than the influence previously exerted by a virus similar in character to that of a fatal anthrax virux? And by what technical term could we more appropriately speak of this influence exerted by a similar virus than by Hahnemann's word: "homoeopathy"?[161]

### (b) Allergology

This is another extensive subject requiring little elaboration by us here. The use of pollen extracts, house-dust extracts, etc. to reduce and eliminate sensitivity to these and other substances is clearly an instance of the application of similars and is recognized as such.

### (c) Use of Drugs According to the Similars Principle

Many drugs are used "homoeopathically" in allopathic medicine today. In other words, they are used to treat conditions whose symptoms are identical with those produced by this drug on a healthy person. Since the same drugs are often employed in homoeopathy for approximately the same conditions, to this extent their allopathic and homoeopathic uses overlap.

Allopathy does not recognize these homoeopathic parallels and hypothesizes various physiological and pathological mechanisms to explain the action of these medicines. Whether or not these "explanations" are scientifically valid, and they vary from one decade to the next in any case, they do not necessarily contradict the homoeopathic law of similars — which is only another way of observing and interpreting the very same phenomena.

Thus conventional medicine relies unconsciously on the homoeopathic law of similars for many of its more effective drugs, although applying this law in a crude way — without the individualization which is a necessity in homoeopathy.

However, the following discussion encompasses a broader area than merely the parallels between the allopathic and homoeopathic uses of drugs. It includes the whole range of phenomena falling under the concepts of "opposite" effects of large and small doses, "paradoxical" effects, etc. — in short, the biphasal action of medicines on the living organism as a function of dose size.

The following examples are only a few of the many which could be mentioned.

*Colchicum*, which has been used since time immemorial in the treatment of gout, produces numerous gout symptoms in its homoeopathic provings: "tingling in right big toe, as if it would go to sleep; pain in left big toe, as if nail would grow into flesh; pain in ball of left big toe, as if inflamed," etc.[162] It is used homoeopathically as one of the remedies for the gout syndrome.

*Colchicum* has also been found useful allopathically in a rare disease known as Familial Mediterranean Fever (Familial Paroxysmal Polyserositis), marked by arthritic joint pains as well as sharp pains in the chest which make breathing difficult.[163] The proving of *Colchicum* has, in addition to the arthritic joint pains, also "violent cutting pain in the chest, interrupting breathing. Lancinating pain, as with a knife, in right side of chest," etc.[164]

The homoeopathic proving of digitalis gives several pages of heart symptoms, including "thready, slow and intermittent pulse. Pulse very slow and weak. Irregular small pulse,"[165] etc. It is the homoeopathicity of digitalis to these heart symptoms which has made it a favorite in certain heart conditions for almost two centuries.[166]

Marijuana has been used in homoeopathy since the mid-nineteenth century. Its provings yield such symptoms as "pressure from back of eyes forwards. Cornea becomes obscured . . . Cornea becomes opaque . . . Cataract."[167] And, of course, there is much discussion today of the curative effect of cannabis in glaucoma and corneal opacity, with the parallel observation that its mode of action is unclear or unknown.[168] In 1900 John Henry Clarke's (homoeopathic) *Dictionary of Practical Materia Medica* was recommending *Cannabis sativa* for "eyes; corneal opacity," on the strength of its provings.[169]

It is known that the IUD with a copper element in it works in some way to prevent conception, presumably because minute quantities of copper leach into the wearer's reproductive system. The proving of *Cuprum metallicum* gives a variety of symptoms for the female reproductive organs, including "spasms," "delayed or suppressed menstruation," "violent cramps,"[170] etc.

In the 1920's a *Belladonna* derivative was discovered by allopathy to be effective, in minute doses, for the treatment of

71

infantile colic. Colic symptoms appear in the provings of *Belladonna*, and it had long been in common use by homoeopaths for treating colic in infants.[171]

The proving of *Rauwolfia serpentina* shows increased blood pressure with irregular heartbeat.[172] Both homoeopathy and allopathy use this substance to reduce blood pressure. Its mental symptoms in the homoeopathic proving include "increased emotional excitability and lability of moods. Alternation of irritability, excitability, and mild depression . . . Inner restlessness," and, of course, allopathic reserpine is used to treat "agitated psychotic states."[173]°

Nitroglycerine was first introduced into medicine by Constantine Hering. He found that the provings yielded a number of cardiac symptoms and used nitroglycerine (known in homoeopathy as *Glonoin*) to treat angina pectoris and other heart conditions.[174] A century later this medicine is used both homoeopathically and allopathically for the management of angina pectoris.

Metallic gold, whose proving yields a series of rheumatic symptoms, and which has been used commonly in homoeopathy for rheumatic complaints, was introduced into allopathy in 1935 by Forestier who observed that gold salts seem to have no direct antibacterial action and must thus operate by stimulating the defense reaction of the host.[175] He tested it, with reported good results, in more than 550 cases of rheumatoid arthritis, and gold salts are still used in allopathy today to treat rheumatoid arthritis and other chronic forms of polyarthritis.[176] Gold preparations have also been used in both allopathy and homoeopathy for the treatment of tuberculosis.[177]

*Veratrum viride*, which in homoeopathic proving yields both increased and decreased pulse rate, is used both homoeopathically and allopathically to treat hypertension.[178]

This medicine has been out of fashion in allopathy recently because the therapeutic dose is too close to the toxic dose. Of course, from the homoeopathic point of view this is an

___

°One reserpine investigator wrote: "although, in the light of our present dosage regime, the 1 mg. given daily verged on the homoeopathic, the results were still conclusive enough to demonstrate that the number of assaults, the number of restraints, and the general noise and disturbance in the ward were all reduced as a result of medication" (*Annals of the New York Academy of Sciences* LXI [1955], Art. 1, 85).

advantage, indicating that the substance has an inherently powerful effect on the organism and thus is a valuable remedy when used skilfully.

The provings of *Stramonium* and *Lobelia* yield many lung symptoms: "extremely difficult breathing caused by a very strong constriction at middle of chest, which impedes respiratory movements," "spasmodic asthma," "excessive sense of suffocation," etc.,[178] and both of these remedies are used to treat asthma in the homoeopathic school. Consequently the use of cigarettes ("Asthmador") made of these substances as inhalent remedies in asthma is homoeopathic. Some years ago the U.S. Food and Drug Administration queried whether Asthmador cigarettes were truly effective in relieving asthma, presumably because the mechanism of action of these substances had not been clarified in the allopathic school but also perhaps because of a lingering feeling that no inexpensive medicine can be really beneficial. As a *Washington Post* columnist noted: "asthma may not be the kind of illness that can be effectively treated by puffing on a jimson-weed cigarette that retails for a nickel."[179]

Ephedrine (from the *Ephedra vulgaris*) also yields a number of asthma symptoms in the homoeopathic proving: "ordinary exertions caused respiration to be wheezing in character," etc.[180] And several allopathic asthma preparations today are based upon ephedrine.

The homoeopathic provings of adrenalin also give rise to asthma symptoms: "sensation of thoracic constriction," "depression of respiratory center," "cough," "expectoration of gelatinous mucus which is hard to detach," etc.[181] And, of course, adrenalin (epinephrin) has been used allopathically to relieve paroxysms of asthma. Because of its biphasal action, however, an overdose will intensify the symptoms this medicine is designed to relieve. In the early 1960's several thousand asthmatics died in England from using adrenalin dispensed in too large a dose from a pressurized aerosol container — probably the greatest epidemic of iatrogenic death in recent history.[182] A homoeopathic physician had warned as early as 1910 that an overdose with the crude drug leads to: "increase of respiratory movements, soon followed by suffocation and death from paralysis of medulla and pneumogastric."[183]

The allopathic anti-coagulant drug, dicumarol, is made

73

from spoiled clover (*Melilotus*) which, in its homoeopathic provings, yields a variety of hemorrhages, especially from the nose and lungs.[184] Consequently, in homoeopathy this drug is used to prevent hemorrhage, and not to prevent blood clotting.[185]

An allopathic experiment demonstrating the law of similars was reported some years ago in the *New England Journal of Medicine*. It involved three substances — caerulein, cholecystokinin, and pentagastrin — known for their ability to stimulate gastric acid secretion. When secretion was stimulated by intravenous administration of pentagastrin, addition of either of the other two substances to the intra-venous drip was found to inhibit secretion rather than (as anticipated) to reinforce the influence of the pentagastrin.[186] In an editorial entitled "Treating Like with Like" the editor noted: "at first glance it might be supposed that gastrin, cholecystokinin, and caerulein, with their identical terminal peptide sequences and overlapping functions, would exert an additive effect if simultaneously released or administered. It has become quite clear, however, that this is not necessarily so; to the contrary, these substances often act antagonistically . . ."[187]

Students of medical history know that ergot of rye — a fungus growing on rye under damp conditions — causes the disease known as St. Anthony's Fire: constriction of the blood vessels, especially in the arms and legs, and progressive gangrene. One historian described this condition: "an icy chill developed in the arms and legs, and this was succeeded by a torturing burning sensation. As though consumed by internal fire, the limbs became black and then shriveled and fell from the body. Some of those afflicted by the disease died, but many recovered, maimed and distorted even by the loss of all their limbs, so that there was left only the trunk and head . . . As late as the eighteenth century the hospital of the Order of St. Anthony in Vienna had a collection of withered and blackened limbs, relics of the afflicted who had received succor there."[188]

The symptoms of ergot poisoning (and, consequently, of the ergot provings) thus include numbness of the hands and arms with loss of sensation, painful swelling, cramps, a burning sensation, contraction of the fingers, etc., and homoeopaths have long used ergot *(Secale cornutum)* to treat gangrene, Raynaud's disease, and circulatory difficulties of various kinds.[189] In 1933 an allopathic physician reported successful treatment of several cases of Raynaud's disease with small doses of ergot, some of the patients manifesting aggravation of the symptoms for a short time after the commencement of therapy.[190] And in the 1940's an ergot-based medicine (hydergine) was introduced into allopathy for the treatment of intermittent claudication and peripheral vascular disease.[191]

The provings of ergot also yield a variety of headaches, and the homoeopathic school pioneered the use of ergot for headaches in the nineteenth century.[192] Today such ergot compounds as methysergide maleate and ergotamine tartrate are used in allopathy to treat migraine and other types of headache.

Even the hallucinatory symptoms of LSD (an ergot derivative) are prefigured in the nineteenth-century homoeopathic provings, and the (allopathic) suggestion that schizophrenia should be treated with LSD is an unsophisticated application of the law of similars.[193]

Snake and insect poisons have a very powerful effect upon the human and animal organism and for that reason were incorporated into homoeopathy at an early stage in its history. One of Hering's first books (in 1837) was on this subject.[194] Some decades later allopathy also came to realize the significance of snake and insect poisons for medicine, and today they are used in both schools.

The homoeopathic proving of rattlesnake venom *(Crotalus horridus)* yields many lung and chest symptoms: "cough with bloody expectoration. Tickling from a dry spot in larynx," etc.[195] Today both schools treat bronchial asthma and upper respiratory tract diseases with rattlesnake venom.[196]

Cobra venom *(Naja tripudians)* has been employed in homoeopathy since the nineteenth century to treat heart muscle damage following infectious disease or a heart attack.[197] A recent publication mentions the allopathic use of a cobra venom fraction to treat myocardial infarction.[198]

The provings of this substance also yield a variety of facial pains: "pain in left temple and in left orbital region, extending to occiput," etc., and both schools use it to treat trifacial neuralgia.[199]

One of the commonest applications of snake poisons is for their effect on the coagulation of the blood. This is biphasal — promoting or inhibiting coagulation depending upon dose size, as was shown by a researcher in 1904. Homoeopaths tend to use these substances for their anticoagulant properties (in phlebitis, thrombophlebitis, etc.), while allopaths seem to use them more for their coagulant properties (in hemorrhages, hemophilia, prevention of Shwartzman's phenomenon, etc.).[201]

The homoeopathic provings of bumble bee venom (*Apis mellefica*) give a number of arthritis and rheumatism symptoms, and bee venom is used to treat arthritis and rheumatism in both schools.[202] Other indications in homoeopathy for the use of bee venom are edema and nephritis, and the allopathic literature also contains reports of the treatment of these conditions with bee venom.[203]

The (allopathic) "side effects" of a drug, representing the long-term poisonous effect of a drug on the patient's organism, are the approximate equivalent of the homoeopathic proving symptoms. Consequently, "side effects" will often indicate the area of application of the medicine. Quinine, for instance, when used for long periods, causes irregularities of the heart beat, and homoeopaths have used quinine for more than a century to treat some cardiac arrhythmias.[204] The use of quinine to treat auricular fibrillation was discovered by allopathy in 1912.[205] Streptomycin was introduced in the mid-1940's for the treatment of tuberculosis and was at once seen to give rise to various ear symptoms: deafness, vertigo, and associated ear noises. This led researchers in both the homoeopathic and allopathic schools, in the late 1940's, to use streptomycin in the treatment of Meniere's disease.[206] The drug, alloxan (mesoxalyl urea), used by allopathic investigators in various nutrition experiments, is known to cause diabetes, and it has been employed successfully by homoeopathic physicians to treat diabetes: glycosuria disappears, and the blood sugar level returns to normal.[207]

Many drugs prescribed in the allopathic treatment of cancer are known to be carcinogenic.[208] The appearance of secondary tumors and cancers in patients undergoing treatment for cancer is thus a striking parallel to the appearance of "super-infections" in patients with bacterial diseases undergoing treatment with anti-bacterial substances. In both cases the "similar" effect of the medicines used intensifies the very condition which is being treated.

While numerous other examples could be given, the above are sufficient to demonstrate that the use of "similars" in homoeopathy can be supported by much empirical evidence from allopathic practice.

The rough parallels between the symptoms from homoeopathic provings and the allopathic disease entities in which these medicines are used should not, of course, be considered an exhaustive analysis of the homoeopathic indications for these remedies. They are only suggestions about the kinds of morbific states in which these drugs may be employed homoeopathically provided the remainder of the patient's symptoms match the drug pathogenesis.

# Chapter Ten
# Hering's Law and Chronic Disease

The concept of chronic disease is extremely important in homoeopathic therapeutic doctrine. Mention has already been made of Hering's Law of the movement of symptoms, and how it governs the relationship between acute and chronic disease as well as between somatic and mental disease. On the basis of their experience with this law and its effects homoeopathic physicians attribute much of today's chronic disease to the indiscriminate allopathic use of medicines which have a suppressive effect on acute conditions and transform them into chronic ones.

The concern of homoeopathic physicians is entirely justified. About one half of the American population suffers from a chronic disease, and over 23 million (about 1 in 9) suffer some impairment of mobility as a consequence.[209]

Of the 23 million whose mobility is impaired, 15.5% have heart disease, 14.1% arthritis or rheumatism, 6.9% an impairment of the back or spine, 6.7% an impairment of the lower extremities or hips, 5% asthma or hay fever, 4.8% a visual impairment, 4.6% hypertension without heart involvement, and 4.4% a mental or nervous condition.[210] To this listing should be added the various kinds of cancer which homoeopathy regards as chronic diseases and which claimed the lives of 350,000 Americans in 1973 and over 400,000 in

1980.[211] By the end of the century about 500,000 Americans are expected to die from cancer every year; one man in five, and one woman in four, will develop this disease.[212]

Various explanations and theories of chronic disease, and its rising incidence, have been propounded by allopathy. But little or no attention has been paid to the possibility that it results in part from the incorrect medical treatment of acute conditions.

As the following passages from the homoeopathic literature indicate, this school holds that the *natural progress and stages* of a patient's illness have to be respected by the physician — at the risk of turning acute conditions into chronic ones:

> I find that very often it is lucky for a patient when his skin remains uncured, that is, not cured at the expense of health . . . skin eruptions are, for Hahnemann, nature's way of quieting an internal disease which threatens vital organs, by developing an external local malady; the object being to keep diseased this non-essential part . . . . In regard to local affections even the popular mind has traditions as to the danger of curing them locally. Many an old woman (in the past, anyway) jealously guarded her "bad leg" because she had, or knew of, the dire consequences following the cure of such an affliction. And has not one been told "he had a rash all over his back before, and when that was cured, his asthma came: he always thought it was that!" So much so that one has got into the habit of asking a new asthma patient, "When did you have an eruption?" "Never," and the next time, "you asked me about an eruption, and I told you I never had it, but now I remember."[213]
>
> Many forms of suppression will be brought out by the homoeopathic remedy, such as the reappearance of skin eruptions suppressed by various ointments, catarrhal complaints, and gonorrhoeal discharges suppressed by injections, followed by rheumatic troubles. Leucorrhoeal discharges stopped by local treatments, followed by ovarian and uterine troubles. Symptoms will disappear in the reverse order of their appearance: that is, under homoeopathic treatment the last symptoms to come are the first to go. . . . The return of old symptoms is one of

79

the best signs that you are really curing your patient and must not be interfered with.[214]

Miss D., 51, had a tumor in left breast for years which continued to grow and become painful. . . . At the first examination I found a hard tumor adherent to the skin in the left breast the size of an apple, with strongly retracted nipple and at times severe burning and stitching pains. For years she had been plagued by facial acne which disappeared a long time ago. This was followed by rapid growth of the then small tumor. . . . She was given a dose of Sulphur 12C every night; her diet was regulated, and the breast covered with cotton. After two months the patient reported that lately the facial acne had returned and that the entire back was covered with acne. The breast pains were much relieved, and the tumor seemed to become smaller. I discontinued Sulphur and regulated the diet. In a month I found the tumor decidedly decreased, and the pain practically gone. During the next month it was reduced to the size of a bean. Today, after 13 years, the patient is still entirely well and never had the slightest recurrence.[215]

The following case illustrates the importance of allowing internal disorders to be discharged through the skin, rather than suppressing them with treatments directed at the skin. It also illustrates the concept of homoeopathic "aggravation" discussed earlier.

About two years ago a man in his forties came to my office. For six months he had made the rounds of dermatologists, visiting 7 or 8 of the best known men in New York and Brooklyn. Lotions, salves, oral medications, and injections had all been tried without result. At all times he wore white cotton gloves because the reddish-brown eruption on both hands emitted a foul odor and watered constantly. At least 3 or 4 daily changes of gloves were necessary, and he feared to approach his clients because of the condition of his hands. . . . He feared loss of his mind and contemplated suicide.

Careful questioning did not reveal any marital discord although he admitted a lack of interest in sex. Venereal disease was denied, both personally and in his family. . . .

In spite of the denial of luetic history and report of negative tests by previous doctors, the patient's exhaustion and emaciation, the mental picture, and the need for alcoholic stimulation, together with the modalities, made me decide on *Syphilinum* as the remedy of choice.°

The patient had never had homoeopathic treatment previously and was therefore warned that the drug he was to receive was a very potent one and might cause him to become much worse within 12 to 36 hours. . . . It was most fortunate that I had so impressed him, for as he related to me a week later, he felt dreadful about 18 hours after taking the remedy. Fluid poured from his hands at such a rate that he could not wear gloves, and the burning became intense. He became frightened and would have sought other attention had he not remembered my telling him that a severe reaction would be followed by a quick cure. After six hours of intense suffering relief set in, and in one week there was hardly any evidence of the dreadful disease he had had. In the almost two years since his recovery there has been no return of symptoms. . . .[216]

Since allopathy is unaware of Hering's .Law and its implications, the literature does not discuss this concept systematically, but, even so, occasional *obiter dicta* can be found which illustrate it.

Tuft wrote in 1931:

In such acute exanthematous diseases as measles, scarlet fever, smallpox, or chickenpox, the presence of a marked skin eruption has always been considered of good prognostic import, and not infrequently when the eruption was scanty, measures were used to bring it out more strongly. . . . Again, in syphilis, it is well known that patients with marked primary or secondary skin manifestations practically never develop nervous or severe visceral involvement and that an arsphenamine dermatitis always appears to offer a favorable prognosis in patients with visceral syphilis. Finally, it is a clinical fact that patients with skin tuberculosis rarely develop pulmonary involvement. These are all evidences of the fact that, in addition to purely

° *Syphilinum* is a remedy prepared from a syphilis chancre.

mechanical protection, the skin also seems to have a specific biological function, designed to protect the internal organs from disease agents. . . . [217]

Zinsser reported in 1939 on "evidence which suggests that by virtue of its chemical composition the skin may possess the function of removing toxic substances introduced into the body . . . this accounts . . . for a variety of dermal reactions such as toxic erythema, urticaria, etc."[218]

The commonly observed association in allopathic practice between gonorrhoea and gonococcal arthritis, or rheumatism and rheumatic heart disease, is also evidence of the operation of Hering's Law. In treating rheumatic fever homoeopaths first endeavor to clear up the heart symptoms. Thereupon the joints become *more* painful and inflamed, but further treatment enables them also to return to normal. James Tyler Kent wrote:

> In cases of rheumatism of the heart you find, if the patient is recovering, that his knees become rheumatic, and he may say: "Doctor, I could walk all over the house when you first came to me, but now I cannot walk, my joints are so swollen." If the doctor does not know that that means recovery, he will make a prescription that will drive the rheumatism away from the feet and knees, and it will go back to the heart, and the patient will die; and it need hardly be stated that the traditional doctor does not know this, as he resorts to this plan as his regular and only plan of treatment, and in the most innocent way kills the patient.[219]

The concepts, "suppression" and "rebound," commonly encountered in the allopathic literature, are further evidence of the truth of Hering's Law.

"Suppression" means that symptoms may disappear while the pathological process continues. Thus a recent work on the treatment of syphilis states: "it is possible that much syphilis is suppressed, but possibly not cured, by the widespread and not always discriminating use of antibiotics."[220] The consequence of such suppression is the development of neurological sequelae in patients treated for syphilis with antibiotics, and this has been suggested in a recent work by Vithoulkas.[221]

But when the medication causing the suppression is

stopped, the symptoms often recur in a more intense and violent fashion than prior to the therapy. This is known as "rebound," and it occurs in many therapeutic situations.

A common effect of the treatment of chronic acid indigestion with alkaline medicines is "acid rebound" — an even higher level of gastric acidity (hence, a common homoeopathic treatment for gastric acidity in the past has been with acid medicines).[222] Use of fluorinated corticosteroids to treat certain skin conditions often leads to "rebound," with intensification of the disease, upon cessation of therapy. Burry wrote in 1973: "Rosacea is suppressed by these steroids only to 'rebound' once they are withdrawn. Further application of the steroid will give symptomatic relief and control the rebound inflammation, leading to prolonged use which promotes and spreads a steroid-induced, rosacea-like entity composed of erythema, edema, pustulation, and telangiectasia."[223] Feinstein wrote about steroid therapy in rheumatic fever: "the rebounds, in all likelihood, represented the clinical appearance of the 'accumulated' inflammatory stimulus whose overt expression had been previously suppressed by the anti-inflammatory treatment."[224] The use of sedatives to calm hyperactive children has the effect of making the children more hyperactive than before, once therapy is stopped.[225]

Thus "suppression" and "rebound" are recognized by allopathy, but its interpretation of these phenomena differs diametrically from that accepted by homoeopathy. Allopathy regards the symptoms as intrinsically harmful, being the external signs of an internal morbific process; hence their suppression is justified, and "rebound" only means a recurrence of the underlying "disease." Homoeopathy, however, regards the symptoms as *in nearly all instances beneficial phenomena:* their suppression thus means suppression of the organism's own self-healing effort. "Rebound," in turn, means the desperate attempt of the body's healing power to assert itself against *both* the "disease" *and* the improper suppressive medicine.

This all brings to mind comments made not long ago by Dickinson W. Richards, a Nobel Prize winner in medicine and professor emeritus of the Columbia University College of Physicians and Surgeons. In discussing the toxic effects of many modern drugs, he asked:

Are we indeed trying to work with nature or are we trying to work against and control it? . . . it would appear that man is moving along rather complacently in the belief that he will one day conquer nature and bring all its forces under his control. Perhaps he will. On the other hand there is increasing evidence that he is not controlling nature at all but only distorting it . . . his powers have extended so far that nature itself, formerly largely protective . . . seems to have become largely retaliatory. Let man make the smallest blunder in his far-reaching and complex physical or physiological reconstructions, and nature, striking from some unforeseen direction, exacts a massive retribution.[226]

Sometimes, however, no "rebound" occurs. While the disease has not been cured, the drugs employed have imposed a new and different form upon the curative efforts of the organism, perverting them into different channels. This is what is called a "drug-induced chronic disease."

The incipient development of this process is seen in the much-discussed "adverse reactions" or "side effects" of therapeutic drugs. The literature of this problem is very extensive and needs no recapitulation by us here. But, while extensive, it does not go far enough. Specifically, as has been noted by Gardner and Cluff, studies of "side effects" and "adverse reactions" do not deal with the "delayed untoward effects of drugs, such as: (1) the role of drugs in the etiology or exacerbation of 'auto-immune' or degenerative diseases, (2) the role of drugs as oncogenic agents, and (3) the effect of drugs on fetal wastage and teratogenicity."[227]

One may logically assume that the long-term, "delayed untoward effects" of the abuse of medicinal drugs are similar to the observed short-term effects. And the typical short-term "side effects" of drugs are the development of tumors and cancers, heart and circulatory difficulties, arthritis and rheumatism, and other degenerative conditions. Hence there is a good *prima facie* case for the belief that the presently observed epidemic of chronic illness in industrialized societies is due, at least in part, to the — also observed — overprescribing of drugs in these same societies. Iatrogenic disease is being converted into chronic disease.

At the very least, the truth of Hering's Law in its relationship to this problem is well worth considering.

Modern discussion of the principal chronic diseases emphasizes the obscurity surrounding their causation:

> With the exception of gout, neither the cause nor cure of chronic joint disability is known.[228]
> There are many theories of the etiology of ulcerative colitis, but few established facts.[229]
> [Bronchitis is] a chronic disease of which the cause is unknown.[230]
> Now, of course, we do not know the cause of [ulcerative colitis and Crohn's Disease]. We are dealing with disorders that have been described as idiopathic or nonspecific, and this terminology reflects our limited knowledge.[231]

About cancer the National Academy of Sciences wrote recently:

> The enormity of our ignorance about cancer receives less emphasis than it merits. Much is said about the lines of research that appear promising today — virology, cellular immunology, and genetics, for example — but too little is made of the genuine possibility that any or all of today's leads . . . could turn out to be wrong leads.[232]

Medical authorities attempt to elucidate the causes of such diseases following traditional paths when a new approach is needed. While investigation along the lines suggested by our analysis above would encounter considerable political opposition within the medical profession, it offers a hope of resolving a major, and growing, problem of twentieth-century medicine.

# Chapter Eleven
# Clinical Evidence in Homoeopathy

Homoeopathy does not make use of the disease entities of allopathy but defines the illness of the given patient in terms of the symptoms from provings. For this reason it is extremely difficult, perhaps impossible, to develop homoeopathic series which would be comparable with the series accepted in allopathy. Nonetheless, homoeopaths have from time to time attempted to develop such series, and a sampling of their efforts is presented here.

### (a) Mixed Series

The earliest recorded publication in homoeopathy of a series of mixed cases was that of Quinton in 1945, who analyzed 100 consecutive cases of nearly as many different "diseases": 8 fibrositis, 6 prostatic ulcers, 6 peptic ulcers, 5 chronic catarrh, 5 chronic migraine, 4 fibroids, 4 hypotension, 3 each of menopausal syndrome, rheumatoid arthritis, obesity, chronic mastitis, cholecystitis, chronic colds, hyperthyroid, tuberculosis, etc. Quinton evaluated his own results as "brilliant" in 6 cases, "good" in 54 cases, "fair" in 32 cases, and "failure" in 8 cases.[233]

Stephenson in 1956 published a comprehensive analysis of 100 consecutive case histories: 6 headaches, 6 rheumatic pain, 6 hemorrhoids, 5 skin rash, 4 asthma, 4 fatigue with insomnia,

3 bronchitis, 3 constipation, 3 obesity, 3 epigastric pain, 3 cholecystitis, 3 genito-urinary infection, and others. He found that one fifth of the cases, by their own account, had at least 50% relief of the complaint; one fourth had less than 25% relief (also by their own account), while the remainder fell somewhere in between.[234]

In 1961 Stephenson published a series of 26 pediatric cases, ranging in age from newborn to 16, with the following complaints: 4 tonsillitis, 3 frequent colds, 3 easily fatigued, 2 sinusitis, 2 sore throats, 2 personality disorders, 1 multiple caries, 1 frequent abdominal pains, 1 strabismus, and 1 ulcerative colitis with a colostomy. By Stephenson's own evaluation the results of treatment were: "excellent" in 4 cases, "good" in 10 cases, "fair" in 3, "poor" in 3, and "unknown" in 6.[235]

It is not easy to determine the significance of these series. Homoeopathic physicians have always maintained that any patient who is curable at all is curable by homoeopathic medicines. Thus, to the extent that the conditions mentioned in the above series are actually curable, the failure rates reported reflect the physician's inability to find the correct medicine. (Of course, no physician should be held to a standard of perfection.)

### (b) Specific "Diseases"

In 1957 Hubbard and Stephenson published their results in 100 consecutive cases of arthralgia, concluding that the majority (all of whom had suffered for at least ten years) obtained subjective relief within one month of treatment. Ninety-two of the patients obtained subjective relief within 6 months. Thirteen obtained objective relief (joint changes) within six months.[236]

McGrath in 1948 reported on 50 cases of vasomotor rhinitis, in which about 18 different medicines were employed. However, he did not indicate the results of treatment.[237]

Stephenson in 1959 reported on 33 consecutive cases of sinusitis treated with a variety of medicines and all in dilutions higher than 30C: one third reported relief within one month; in 1963 he presented 17 consecutive allergy cases from one month's practice, all of whom responded to treatment.[238]

In 1958 Redfield and Stephenson reported on 35 consecutive cases of duodenal ulcer. All received the same drug —

*Anacardium orientale* — in dilutions lower than 30C, and about three fourths responded to treatment within one month.[239]

Patel in 1973 discussed 100 cases of asthma in children. All were treated with *Luffa operculata*. Thirty-six had relief for 1-3 months, 26 for 3-6 months, 11 for 6-9 months, and 10 for 9-12 months.[240]

In 1958 Hubbard reported on 51 consecutive cases of headache. More than two thirds reported relief within one month, even in cases where the headache had been present for more than ten years; in the same year Stephenson reported on 28 consecutive cases of headache with the same results.[241] All patients of both physicians received medicines in dilutions higher than 30C.

In 1957 Hubbard and Stephenson presented 86 consecutive cases of eczema. About half obtained relief within one month of commencing treatment, the relief lasting for one to three months.[242]

In 1966 Stewart reported on 40 consecutive patients with heart disease at the Glasgow Homoeopathic Hospital, treated with a number of different medicines. He did not analyze the results.[243]

In 1973 Mossinger presented a discussion of 18 cases of cysts treated with *Silica*. He concluded that there was a 95% probability that two thirds of the cysts would disappear within 4-8 months of commencing treatment.[244]

In 1980 a group of allopathic and homoeopathic physicians in Glasgow investigated the effect of homoeopathic treatment in rheumatoid arthritis. Forty-six patients meeting the criteria of the American Rheumatism Association for definite rheumatoid arthritis were treated, half with conventional anti-inflammatory medications together with (homoeopathic) placebo and half with conventional anti-inflammatory medications together with the indicated homoeopathic remedies. None of the patients knew that the trial involved homoeopathic preparations, and the trial was double-blind in that neither physicians nor patients knew who was receiving placebo and who was receiving the homoeopathic preparations. The patients on homoeopathic remedies showed significant improvement over those on placebo, as measured by change in articular index, limbering up time, grip strength, pain, and functional index, the authors observing:

> The results of this trial confirm the impression . . . that homoepathic treatment is effective in the control of patients with rheumatoid arthritis. . . . It would . . . seem that the differences observed were due to the remedies administered and not to any psychological relationship between patient and physician or to placebo response to the homoeopathic substances. The fact that neither placebo group improved significantly is strong evidence that it is the drug and not the doctor which is effective.[245]

Furthermore, these results duplicated those obtained from an earlier pilot study.[246]

The same observation may be made about these various series as about the earlier ones. When only one medicine is used, the results cannot be considered to demonstrate anything valid about homoeopathy, since the *sine qua non* of homoeopathic practice is selection of the remedy to match the totality of the patient's symptoms. This precludes any prescription of a remedy in function of the patient's "disease." Those series in which a variety of remedies were prescribed are closer to the spirit of homoeopathy, but failures of treatment should still be ascribed to improper selection of the remedy, and not to any inherent "unreliability" of the homoeopathic prèparations themselves, since they always have the desired effect when prescribed correctly.

The Glasgow trial is particularly interesting in being the first homoeopathic-allopathic collaborative trial since the mid-nineteenth century (also the first to be reported in an allopathic journal). The homoeopathic results would have been even better if the patients had not been receiving anti-inflammatory drugs at the same time, since these are known to counteract homoeopathic preparations. In the pilot study, which lasted for a year, it was possible to discontinue all conventional therapy in 42% of the patients.

It remains to be seen if the allopathic profession will understand the significance of these results.

Finally, mention may be made of an experiment conducted in England during the Second World War on human volunteers to determine the efficacy of homoeopathic medicines in preventing and treating the effects of mustard gas. A 2 mm. drop of a 10% solution of mustard gas provided by the Ministry of Home Security was applied to the forearms of 127 subjects. Another 113 persons were used as controls. A 30C potentiation of mustard gas given preventively was found to inhibit development of the lesion. A 30C potentiation of *Rhus toxicodendron* (poison ivy) applied curatively was found to have the same effect.[247]

### (c) Homoeopathic Veterinary Medicine

The use of homoeopathy in veterinary medicine is of particular interest because the psychosomatic factor in treatment is largely excluded.

In 1945 Cross presented several cases of treatment of pruritus and furuncles in dogs (mostly with ultramolecular dilutions).[248]

Bardoulat published a book in 1949 on the treatment of pyelonephritis, nephritis, nephritic colic, urinary lithiasis, essential haematuria, cystitis, urethritis, anuria, and ulcerous balanitis in farm animals, using 3C, 4C, 5C, 6C, and 7C potencies.[249]

Plantureux in 1950 published reports of his experiments in preventing and treating rabies in dogs with microdilutions of rabies virus and such medicines as *Lachesis* (poison of the bushmaster) and *Belladonna*. While the experiments in preventive immunization and preventive treatment after infection were not conclusive, the author obtained 35 cures (33 with injected rabies and 2 with natural rabies). The report does not state the number of animals participating, but, since rabies is regarded as incurable, the results are of interest.[250]

Bardoulat in 1961 reported on trials of 5C, 7C, and 10C microdilutions of diphtheria toxin in treating avian diphtheria. In 8 sets of observations on as many flocks of chickens, he concluded that the diseased birds healed in about 12 days and that the disease did not spread to the remainder of the flock.[251]

MacLeod in 1972 reported on the treatment of pulmonary emphysema, bovine mastitis, bowel edema, vibrionic dysentery, and enteric colibacillosis in different farm animals, using remedies from the lowest to the highest potencies.[252] In another article he presented his treatment for infertility in cows, horses, sheep, dogs, and cats.[253]

Campbell in 1975 described an interesting series of cases,

consisting of three litters (a total of 5 pups) from the same mother guinea pig. All were infected with an eye disease at birth; the pup treated with chloramphenicol became almost blind in that eye, while the 4 pups treated homoeopathically recovered completely.[254]

Finally, as a curiosity, mention may be made of an account by a lion-tamer of his treatment of young lions with teething problems:

> Teething, including that part of the nutrition cycle connected with teething, is the single greatest difficulty in rearing lions in captivity, and I have experimented for many years and evolved what I think is almost foolproof medication. The means used are homoeopathic . . . if a young lion is given, twice daily, two crushed pills of *Calcarea carbonica* [calcium carbonate], *Calcarea phosphorica* [calcium phosphate], and *Silica* in 3X strength, it will have effortless dentition and a bone structure at maximum, having reference to its genetic inheritance.[255]

### (d) The Serum Flocculation Test

The serum flocculation test, as a technique for selecting the "similar" remedy, was developed by George Russell Henshaw, M.D.

After examining and questioning the patient, the physician decides on several remedies which appear more or less to match the patient's symptoms. The serum flocculation test is designed to facilitate the physician's selection of the one "most similar" medicine out of this group.

The apparently indicated remedies are placed in vials to which is added physiologic saline solution (1 cc.). Then .5 cc. of this solution is placed in a second vial to which is added about 2 cc. of serum from the patient (previously centrifuged and diluted). Three possible reactions will then take place on the plane of contact between the saline solution and the patient's blood serum: 1) a distinct heavy base at the plane of contact with a lighter area rising up through the serum, 2) the same distinct heavy base with the area above of equal density, 3) a distinct precipitate at the line of contact which widens in a downward direction. The first of these indicates the similar remedy, while the others represent varying departures from "similarity" with the patient's symptoms.[256]

The serum flocculation test has been used by a number of homoeopathic physicians and apparently with success.

# Chapter Twelve
# Conclusion: Homoeopathy and Scientific Method

The preceding pages have shown that there exists a considerable area of overlap between the principles of homoeopathy and the ideas and practices accepted by conventional allopathic medicine. At the same time, the differences between the two systems are great, and it is well to draw attention to them, if only to throw light on the reasons for the continuing allopathic incomprehension of homoeopathy.

The principal difference is that homoeopathy is a precisely structured doctrine. Even though most of its ideas find their parallels in allopathy, it differs from the latter in that the homoeopathic ideas are mutually consistent and coherent. Whatever is not compatible with these ideas is excluded from homoeopathy. In this discipline medicines may not be prescribed otherwise than in conformity with Hahnemann's three rules.

While these physicians resort to surgery, give dietary instruction, and may employ acupuncture or manipulation, they do not recognize other principles of pharmacological prescribing as compatible with homoeopathy.

Allopathy, in contrast, lacks a precisely defined and delineated set of ideas. It accepts concepts, principles, and procedures from any number of sources, with the result that the various parts of allopathic doctrine are at times inconsistent, and even incompatible, with one another (for instance, the symptom in allopathy is sometimes regarded as beneficial, sometimes as harmful, and no justification or explanation is given for this arbitrary division). As was noted at the outset, in allopathy "the basic laws of health and disease" have not yet been disclosed. "No discipline can claim a greater array of equipment by which its research is carried on, yet none is inferior to [allopathic] medicine in organizing its knowledge into coherent principles."

The precision and rigor of homoeopathy make it harder to practice than the more diffuse allopathy. The homoeopathic physician has little leeway in his selection of the patient's prescription; he must at all times be guided by the symptoms, and if he chooses a wrong remedy, it will usually have no effect.

These difficulties of practice, about which the homoeopaths themselves have often complained and which even led to a split in the homoeopathic profession in the late nineteenth century,[257] make this therapeutic system less attractive to the ordinary physician — who feels that it restricts his freedom and creativity. Therefore, although the homoeopathic profession is a well-entrenched minority in most countries, and has a large and devoted following of patients, it seems unlikely ever to become a majority of the medical profession anywhere.

It is paradoxical that allopathy — which sees itself as searching for the ultimate laws of sickness and health, i.e., for the knowledge which will make medical practice scientific and hence rigorous — should reject the homoeopathic claim to possess this knowledge.

The reason for this rejection is that a rigorously structured medical discipline is burdensome for the practitioner in imposing limitations on his freedom of action (hence the assumed goal of allopathic research — to establish a firm and unwavering structure of cause-and-effect relations to serve as an infallible guide to the practitioner — will never be attained but, like the mirage that it is, will continually recede into the future).

Of course, the allopathic majority is unable to admit (or even recognize) this largely subconscious motive for its hostility to homoeopathy, and instead it relies on the accusation that homoeopathy is "unscientific."

This raises the issue of the true meaning of scientific method in medicine. Much has been written on it elsewhere°, and we will limit ourselves to a few general remarks.

While the allopathic argument against homoeopathy has never been formulated clearly and comprehensively (one of the odder aspects of the 175 years of conflict between the two systems), from the occasional critical pieces appearing here and there one can see that the principal bone of contention is homoeopathy's lack of a physiological-pathological-pharmacological theory. Homoeopaths do not follow the ordinary allopathic technique of first defining an internal pathophysiological process and then selecting a remedy for its supposed capacity to counteract or otherwise influence this patho-physiological process. Instead, they base their selection of remedies exclusively on the symptoms in the provings.

Some examples will make this contrast clear.

We have already noted that both homoeopaths and allopaths use colchicum in gout, digitalis and nitroglycerine in heart conditions, and gold compounds in rheumatism. While the former base these uses on the provings (and hence feel that the allopaths are unconsciously relying on the law of similars), the allopaths themselves justify these applications in terms of prevailing pathological and pharmacological theory:

> Colchicine inhibits migration of granulocytes to the inflammatory area and reduces the increased lactic acid production associated with phagocytosis. By these and possibly other effects on leukocytes colchicine interrupts the cycle of urate crystal deposition and inflammatory response that sustains the acute attack.°°[258]
>
> The main pharmacodynamic property of digitalis is its ability to increase the force of myocardial contraction . . . a positive inotropic action . . . by increasing the rate at which tension or force is developed.[259]

°See the author's *Divided Legacy: A History of the Schism in Medical Thought.* Three volumes (Washington, D.C.: Wehawken Book Co., 1973-1977). Also, Harris L. Coulter, *Homoeopathic Medicine* (St. Louis: Formur, 1975).

°°And yet a case is reported where gouty arthritis was cured with colchicine even though the synovial fluid contained virtually no leucocytes (R. Wade Ortel and David S. Newcombe, "Acute Gouty Arthritis and Response to Colchicine in the Virtual Absence of Synovial-Fluid Leucocytes," *New England Journal of Medicine,* 290 (June 13, 1974), 1363-1364.

The basic pharmacological action of nitrites is to relax smooth muscle . . . nitrite produces a more sustained dilatation of the larger coronary vessels, as determined by arteriography in man . . . the myocardial ischemia associated with coronary artery disease and particularly with attacks of angina pectoris results in decreased lactate extraction or actual net lactate production by the myocardium . . . nitroglycerine can normalize the lactate and potassium gradients. This reflects a decrease in ischemia.[260]

Most drugs used in the treatment of polyarthritis have been anti-inflammatories . . . Recourse to an additional parameter of activity — i.e., ability to influence lysosomal enzymes which, via their cleavage products, give rise to new antigens — has shown that gold salts, for example, which do not belong to the category of classic anti-inflammatory agents, exert an up to 100% inhibitory effect on lysosomal enzymes and are thus able to interrupt at a particular stage the process of auto-immunization.[261]

Clearly allopathy holds that the duty of pharmacological science is to elucidate the cause-and-effect relationship between the remedy and the patient's physiological or pathological condition. Homoeopathy just as clearly avoids cause-and-effect explanations and interprets the action of a medicine on the organism in terms of the more general law of similars.

In a sense, the two "explanations" are not mutually exclusive, at least at this level. Thus, gold compounds do give rise to certain rheumatic symptoms in the provings, and they may also very well "exert an up to 100% inhibitory effect on lysosomal enzymes." But for certain practical, as well as theoretical, reasons the homoeopaths prefer their mode of "explanation" to the allopathic one.

To start with the practical advantages, the homoeopaths consider that their provings permit the development of a large body of information about each medicinal substance, the law of similars enabling the practitioner to apply this knowledge directly to the needs of the particular patient. They ask: if these medicines can be employed with great accuracy purely on the basis of the provings, why is it necessary to resort to theoretical "explanations" which, as is generally admitted, are unreliable and subject to continual change?

Thus the homoeopaths feel that the *reliability* of the information developed in the provings is a great practical advantage. This information has been in steady use for about 175 years without requiring substantial revision. In contrast, allopathic theories change from decade to decade and year to year. How can they be considered reliable?

Thus homoeopathy considers its own approach to be eminently practical, since the information from provings is precise, concrete, and reliable.

Homoeopathy prefers its own approach on more general theoretical grounds as well.

It feels that allopathy's interpretation of medical science as a body of causal relations is outmoded. This reductionist view was accepted in all sciences until the early nineteenth century but has now been discarded by everyone except the allopathic physicians.

And it is perhaps time to discard it here as well. As Rene Dubos stated some years ago:

> The reductionist approach, which has come to dominate so much of medical science, is not sufficient to deal with the complex situations created by the response of men or animals to the administration of biologically active substances.[262]

Needed is a medical science whose postulates and structure resemble those of the other sciences, eschewing "causal" explanations in favor of general hypotheses and laws which describe the behavior of the phenomena and permit prediction.

Homoeopathy meets the formal requirements of such a science and is thus a more up-to-date formulation than allopathy. Its principles and postulates are a coherent body of knowledge describing the behavior of the organism in sickness and health and prescribing the method which must be followed to bring it from sickness to health.

And, as already noted, the greater rigor and precision of the homoeopathic principles would suggest that this discipline is the more "scientific" of the two.

Using the language of scientific method we can say that the homoeopathic principles, together with the detailed rules of their application, constitute a unified hypothesis. When the

97

homoeopathic physician treats a patient according to these principles and rules, he is testing the validity of the hypothesis that cure is through similars. The observed successes of this mode of treatment serve as provisional confirmation of the truth of the homoeopathic hypothesis.

Of course, no hypothesis in science is ever proven correct once and for all, as new evidence may always emerge to contradict or refute the hypothesis. However, to date such contradictory evidence has not come forward, and the provisional truth of the homoeopathic hypothesis is accepted by all who have had experience with it.

It is not possible to test in the same way the correctness of the allopathic "principles" or "rules of application," because none exist. No allopathic "theory" has ever been explicitly formulated, although bits and pieces of one can be found implicit in the allopathic assumptions and underlying allopathic procedures.° Thus the allopathic view of medical science — as a body of cause-and-effect relations — is not only outmoded from the purely formal standpoint, it has never even been adequately developed as an operational theory governing medical practice. A number of trenchant criticisms have been launched against it by homoeopathic and by allopathic thinkers.

In general, the allopathic "causal" explanations often confuse the ascription of causes with the description of mechanisms. What is presented as the pinpointing of a cause turns out to be merely the description of an intermediate mechanism dependent upon a still unknown and concealed cause. The examples given above "explaining" the action of colchicine, digitalis, nitrites, and gold salts all suffer from this defect, and one wonders if *all* such "explanations" will not be equally defective. As Goodman and Gilman have pointed out, "the more a presumed action is studied, the more likely it is to become an effect, and the real action retreats beyond our present means of discovery."[263]

Even as "descriptions of mechanisms" the allopathic formulations are unsatisfactory and inconclusive, often relying ultimately on vague references to the central nervous system to supply missing links in the causal chain.

°The author is working on a critical study of allopathic "theory."

In truth, the incredible complexity of the body's physiology makes all such would-be cause-and-effect explanations seem highly simplistic. A recent allopathic text on drug design states that the effect of a drug on the organism can be divided into: its chemical or molecular action and, then, the chain reaction through the body's other levels of organization: molecular systems, polymolecular systems, cellular systems, polycellular or tissue systems, polytissue or organ systems, etc. With respect to the chemical or molecular effect of the medicine this author observes: "The relation between the constitutional and chemobiodynamically potential aspects of molecules in terms of the first level of chemobiodynamic action is only beginning to be understood[264] . . . ." And he goes on to note that even possession of this chemical or molecular knowledge would not tell the investigator anything about higher-level reactions, since these are determined by the organizational charac-teristics of the higher-level aggregates:

A crucial problem for chemobiodynamics, in the light of the complexity and functional integrity of biologic systems, is the assessment of the potency of drugs in regard to their primary effects. This is a difficult problem, because the existence of many feedback mechanisms often tends either to nullify or to exaggerate responses to a drug. It is of course possible to isolate or insulate various systems making up the biologic system from one another by various means, in order to assess the magnitude of primary or immediate secondary drug effects. These methods require the use of surgical procedures or the blockade of various processes by chemicals whose actions are already fairly well understood. In any case, the experimental details and labor involved, as well as the control procedures that are necessary, are enormous . . . [265]

Even if such a mechanism could be isolated, could it be applied reliably to a single individual patient? Allopathic clinical and physiological research relies upon results achieved

---

°A 1963 text had stated: "I think it is fair to say that we do not know as yet with certainty in specific detail how molecules of *any* drug affect those of *any* cell," but some progress may have been made since that time (see Max Rinkel, *Specific and Non-Specific Factors in Psychopharmacology* [New York: Philosophical Library, 1963], 72).

with groups of animals or groups of patients. As was observed by Bradford Hill, a pioneer in the elaboration of statistical methods in medicine: "Individuals are not necessarily equivalent. It is a group reaction that is under study."[266] But the physician, as opposed to the public health scientist, deals with individuals, not groups, and this gives rise to a severe methodological difficulty:

> The statistical analysis and descriptions usually employed tell us little of a sufficiently predictive nature about the probable response of a given individual within the group. Yet the latter is one of the most challenging problems of biology and *the* most pressing problem of the physician, whose concern is with the individual.[267]

Allopathy looks to the normal or average individual as its standard, but the normal individual does not even exist. The biochemist, Roger Williams, has written:

> Each individual has a distinctive "metabolic pattern," as reflected, for example, in the distinctive composition of his saliva, urine, and blood . . . Such patterns are mirrored very imperfectly by any set of measurements we are now able to make; they are much more deeply rooted than their observed outward manifestations might suggest . . . the differences between the patterns of two normal individuals may be large and of far more than academic interest.[268]

And "the probable connection between variations in drug responses and biochemical individuality has not been generally recognized."[269] Response to drugs is affected by a whole series of factors: (1) species and strain variability, (2) age of the subject and presence of disease, (3) environmental factors such as climate, altitude, season, temperature, time of day, (4) the subject's nutritional status, (5) his previous history, training, and experience, and, finally, his (6) constitution or temperament:

> Constitutional factors also affect the drug response. An individual exhibits in general or in particular a vigor or a feebleness, a susceptibility or insusceptibility to environmental influences, a readiness or lack of self-defense, a

100

completeness or insufficiency of self-repair, which cannot be located in any organ, tissue, or plasma. However obscure in character and origin, such constitutional factors must be recognized and considered . . . These characteristics have been shown to be under genetic control, and the literature is replete with references to temperament and personality as important variables affecting the qualitative and quantitative response to drugs.[270]

Despite these theoretical and practical obstacles, allopathic medicine remains intensely committed to causal explanations. While a technique is occasionally justified in terms of its outcome alone:

The significance of each immunologic event in immunotherapy is not yet clearly defined, nor is the interrelationship of the various parameters understood. Even in the absence of a clear definition of immunologic function, clinicians throughout the world feel that injection therapy is an effective procedure.[271]

In the overwhelming majority of instances a theoretical justification is demanded. *Therapeutic procedures are legitimated in allopathy by being provided with causal explanations.*°

Homoeopathy takes a different approach, assuming that a well-founded practice is its own justification and can dispense with support from ever-changing pathophysiological and pharmacological theory. The absence of any fundamental change in homoeopathic practice over the past 180 years is taken by these physicians to show that the practice was good at the outset.

Thus homoeopathy justifies practice by practice. The provings are pure experiments, and no attempt is made to

---

°One of the main functions of medical theory is thus to furnish the physician with reasons and explanations for the procedures he applies when treating his patients. Lewis Thomas writes that the physician of his father's generation "first of all . . . was expected to walk in and take over. And second, and this was probably the most important of his duties, he had to explain what had happened, and, third, what was likely to happen" (Lewis Thomas, "The Right Track," *Wilson Quarterly*, Spring, 1980, 90). Theory is structured in the form of cause-effect relationships in order to fulfill the social function of legitimating the physician's therapeutic procedures. This is as true today as a generation ago, if only because the physician must justify his failures.

"explain" why a given medicine yields a given symptom pattern. Homoeopathic doctrine is not, and can never be, a theory of physiology or of the intimate effects of drugs on the organism. It is a set of precise rules for practice. It is the crystallized practice of the generations of physicians who have applied and developed the hypothesis proposed by Hahnemann and expanded by Hering and Kent.

By rejecting physiological theory as a guide to medical practice homoeopathy avoids many of the problems encountered by allopathy. As already noted, these stem in part from the conflict in allopathy between the theory, derived from experience with groups, and the practice, which is necessarily with individuals. Homoeopathy's elaborate symptomatic descriptions permit an extreme degree of individualization in case-taking — on the basis of a rigorous method — and eliminate the necessity of regarding the patient as merely the representative of a pathological category.

Homoeopathy rejects the allopathic belief that the mechanisms of medicinal substances can be ultimately explained. The "real action" of a drug will *always* retreat beyond the investigator's means of discovery if it is sought at the cellular, molecular, or sub-molecular level, since mechanisms at all of these levels are determined by the behavior of the organism *as a whole*.

When the whole body is seen to be the cause of all the changes occurring in it, and it is realized that the behavior of the whole body can be understood through the visible symptoms, the "real action" of the medicine will then be seen to lie on the surface, available to the physician's perception and intelligence.

In this sense homoeopathy is the model of a holistic medical doctrine, and at this time of search for the true meaning of a holistic therapeutics homoeopathy is steadily coming to the fore.

o    o    o

Homoeopathy was singularly unfortunate to emerge in the nineteenth century—when the pervasive engineering and scientific advances enshrined reductionist thinking in the investigation of nature. As a unique form of holistic medicine homoeopathy naturally met with incomprehension from physicians trained in the belief that reductionism was the only true method in science.

Many of the homoeopaths themselves failed to understand the reason for the intellectual gulf between themselves and their allopathic colleagues.

Today the intellectual atmosphere in science is different. Reductionism is seen to be an inadequate method in all other scientific disciplines, and only the large intellectual, emotional and economic investment in this mode of thought perpetuates reductionism in medicine.

At the same time, voices can be heard in allopathic medicine today calling for a reevaluation of its approach and method. Homoeopathy offers itself as an answer to those persons who seek a break with the past and an unprecedented flowering of therapeutic thought in the future.

# References

[1]Ian Stevenson, M.D., "Why Medicine is Not a Science." *Harpers* (April, 1949).

[2]S. Solis-Cohen and T. S. Githens, *Pharmacotherapeutics* (N.Y. and London: Appleton, 1928), 37.

[3]Hans Selye, *The Stress of Life*, Revised Edition (New York: McGraw-Hill, 1978), 358.

[4]*Ibid.*, 55.

[5]*Ibid.*, 336.

[6]*Ibid.*, 62.

[7]W. H. Perkins, *Cause and Prevention of Disease* (Philadelphia: Lea and Febiger, 1938), 23.

[8]Karl Menninger, "Changing Concepts of Disease," *Annals of Internal Medicine* 29 (1948), 318-325, at 324-325.

[9]W. A. Sodeman and W. A. Sodeman, Jr., *Pathologic Physiology* (Philadelphia: Saunders, 1967), 5.

[10]Selye, *op. cit.*, 321.

[11]*Ibid.*, 12.

[12]*Ibid.*, 13.

[13]Hans Zinsser, John F. Enders, and LeRoy D. Fothergill, *Immunity* (New York: Macmillan, 1939), 1-2, 20-22.

[14]Rene J. Dubos, *Bacterial and Mycotic Infections of Man*, Third Edition (Philadelphia: Lippincott, 1958), v, 14.

[15]W. T. Vaughan, "A Theory Concerning the Mechanism and Significance of the Allergic Response," *Journal of Laboratory and Clinical Medicine* 21 (1935-1936), 629-649, at 632.

[16]Selye, *op.cit.*, 38.

[17]J. L. Achord, ed., *Chronic Inflammatory Bowel Disease* (Medcom Press, 1974), 94.

[18]Kathleen J. Deighton, "Cancer — A Systemic Disease with Local Manifestations," *Medical Hypotheses* I:2 (March-April, 1975), 37-40, at 37.

[19]G. Zajicek, "Cancer as a Systemic Disease," *Medical Hypotheses* IV (1978), 193-207, at 193.

[20]*Loc. cit.*

[21]Alexis Carrel, *Man, the Unknown* (New York: MacFadden, 1961), 139

[22]A professor in a British medical school, quoted in T. R. Waugh, "The Trend of Modern Pathology," *Journal of the American Institute of Homoeopathy* 25 (1932), 1141-1147.

[23]F. P. Gay, *Agents of Disease and Host Resistance* (Springfield: Thomas, 1935), 255.

[24]Selye, *op.cit.*, 131 ff.

[25]Solis-Cohen and Githens, *op. cit.*, 22.

[26]Selye, *op. cit.*, 65.

[27]Vaughan, *op. cit.*, 639-640.

[28]*Ibid.*, 631.

[29]Zinsser *et al.*, *op. cit.*, 432.

[30]Noel R. Rose, Felix Milgrom, and Carel J. Van Oss, *Principles of Immunology* (New York: Macmillan, 1973), 4.

[31]Cyril MacBride, ed., *Signs and Symptoms: Applied Pathologic Physiology and Clinical Interpretation*. Fifth Edition (Philadelphia: Lippincott, 1970), 1.

[32]*Ibid.*, 35.

[33]Linn J. Boyd, *A Study of the Simile in Medicine* (Ann Arbor: University of Michigan, 1936), 335. Karl Koetschau, "The Type Effect Hypothesis as a Scientific Basis for the Simile Principle," *Journal of the American Institute of Homeopathy* 23 (1930), 972-1046.

[34]Joseph Wilder, M.D., "The Law of Initial Value in Neurology and Psychiatry: Facts and Problems," *J. Nervous and Mental Disease* 125 (1957) 73-86, at 73. See, also, Joseph Wilder, *Stimulus and Response: the Law of Initial Value* (Bristol, Wright, 1967).

[35]*Loc. cit.*

[36]Selye, *op. cit.*, 334.

[37]Wilder, *op. cit.*, 74.

[38]W. W. Duke, "Variation in the Platelet Count. Its Cause and Clinical Significance," *Journal of the American Medical Association* 65 (1915), 1600-1606, at 1603.

[39]W. Buecherl and E. Buckley,*Venomous Animals and Their Venoms*. Three Volumes (New York and London: Academic Press, 1971), II, 14.

[40]A. B. Searle, *The Use of Colloids in Health and Disease* (London: Constable, 1920), 96.

[41]W. Wolf, *Endocrinology in Modern Practice*. Second Edition (Philadelphia: Saunders 1939), 26-27.

[42]W. Seiffert, "Die Grundlagen der Chemotherapie," *Klinische Wochenschrift* 7 (1928), I, 1497-1502.

[43]Almroth E. Wright, *Studies on Immunization*. First Series (London: Heinimann, 1943), 170.

[44]Alexander Fleming, *Chemotherapy, Yesterday, Today, and Tomorrow* (Cambridge: University Press, 1946), 26.

[45]L. P. Garrod, "The Reactions of Bacteria to Chemotherapeutic Drugs," *British Medical Journal* (1951), i, 205-210.

[46]Hans Eppinger, "Ueber Kollapszustaende," *Wiener Klinische Wochenschrift* 47 (1934), 47-50.

[47]*Journal of the American Medical Association* 174 (1960), 443.

[48]Duke, *op. cit.*, 1603.

[49]N. B. Taylor and C. B. Weld, "A Study of the Action of Irradiated Ergosterol and of its Relationship to Parathyroid Function," *Journal of the Canadian Medical Association* 25 (1931), 20-34, at 34.

[50]Privy Council. Medical Research Council. *Medical Uses of Radium. Summary of Reports from Research Centers for 1931* (London: Published by His Majesty's Stationery Office, 1932), 32-33.

[51]IAEA, *Radiation and Radioisotopes Applied to Insects of Agricultural Importance* (Vienna, 1963), 371.

[52]G. C. LaBrecque, D. W. Meifert, and Carroll N. Smith, "Mating Competitiveness of Chemosterilized and Normal Male House Flies," *Science* 136 (May 4, 1962), 388-389.

[53]Wilder, *op. cit.*, 77.

[54]*Loc. cit.*

[55]*Loc. cit.*

[56]*Loc. cit.*

[57]*Ibid.*, 78.

[58]B. J. Sahakian and T. W. Robbins, "Are the Effects of Psychomotor Stimulant Drugs on Hyperactive Children Really Paradoxical?" *Medical Hypotheses* III:4 (July-August, 1977), 154-158.

[59]Wilder, *op. cit.*, 79.

[60]*Ibid.*, 83.

[61]*Ibid.*, 76.

[62]*Ibid.*, 84.

[63]Max Rinkel, *Specific and Non-Specific Factors in Psychopharmacology* (New York: Philosophical Library, 1963), 72.

[64]USDHEW, *Report of the Conference on the Use of Stimulant Drugs in the Treatment of Behaviorally Disturbed Young School Children*. Washington, D.C., January 11-12, 1971, at 4.

[65]Robert G. Schnackenberg, "Caffeine as a Substitute for Schedule II Stimulants in Hyperkinetic Children," *American Journal of Psychiatry* 130 (1973), 796-798.

[66]P. F. D'Arcy and J. P. Griffin, *Iatrogenic Diseases* (Oxford: at the University Press, 1972), 109.

[67]Starling and Lovatt Evans, *Principles of Human Physiology*, 14th edition (London, J. & A. Churchill, 1968), 1492.

[68]Julius A. Howell, "Silver Nitrate vs. Sulfamylon in the Treatment of Burns," *North Carolina Medical Journal* 29 (1968), 280-283.

[69]Emil Grubbe, "X-Ray Treatment: Its Introduction to Medicine," *Journal of the American Institute of Homeopathy* 39 (1946), 419-422. Grubbe's hand became blistered from overexposure to X-rays during the course of his experiments, and this led one of the professors at the homoeopathic college to suggest its therapeutic use in similar conditions.

[70]Alexander Fleming, *op.cit.* 16.

[71]Linn J. Boyd, *op. cit.*, 250-251.

[72]"Quinine" in *Encyclopedia Britannica*, 1957.

[73]T. D. Luckey, "Antibiotic Action in Adaptation," *Nature* 198 (1963), 263-265.

T. D. Luckey, "Hormoligosis in Pharmacology," *Journal of the American Medical Association* 173 (1960), 44-48. T. D. Luckey, "Modes of Action of Antibiotics in Growth Stimulation," *Recent Progress in Microbiology* (VII International Congress for Microbiology, 1958). T. D. Luckey, "Stimulation of *Turbatrix aceti* by Antibiotics," *Proceedings of the Society for Experimental Biology and Medicine* 113 (1963), 121, 124. T. D. Luckey, "Insecticide Hormoligosis," *Journal of Economic Entomology* 61 (1968), 7-12.

[74]James Stephenson, "The Need for Provings of the Chemical Elements," *Journal of the American Institute of Homeopathy* 50 (1957), 265.

[75]T. F. Allen, *Encyclopedia of Pure Materia Medica* (New York and Philadelphia: Boericke and Tafel, 1874-1880), V, 17.

[76]William Boericke, *Materia Medica with Repertory*. Ninth edition (Philadelphia: Boericke and Tafel, 1927), 475-478.

[77]A. W. Blyth, *Poisons, their Effects and Detection*. Fifth edition (London: Griffin, 1920), 338.

[78]William Boericke, *op. cit.*, 7-11.

[79]A. W. Blyth, *op. cit.*, 377.

[80]William Boericke, *op. cit.*, 110-115.

[81]A. W. Blyth, *op. cit.*, 394.

[82]Samuel Hahnemann, "Was sind Giften, was sind Arzneien?" [What are poisons, what are medicines?], *Journal der practischen Heilkunde* XXIV (1806), st. III, 40-57.

[83]L. U. Gardner, "The Similarity in the Lesions Produced by Silica and by the Tubercle Bacillus," *American Journal of Pathology* 13 (1937), 13-23, at 13.

[84]Michael Mason and H. L. F. Curry, *An Introduction to Clinical Rheumatology*. Second Edition (Tunbridge Wells, Kent: Pitman Medical, 1975), 115.

[85]Guy Beckley Stearns, "Experimental Data on One of the Fundamental Claims in Homoeopathy," *Journal of the American Institute of Homoeopathy* 18 (1925), 433-444, 790-792.

[86]Harris L. Coulter, *Divided Legacy: A History of the Schism in Medical Thought*. Three Volumes (Washington, D.C.: Wehawken Book Co., 1973-1977), III, 490.

[87]Howard P. Bellows, *The Test Drug-Proving of the O. O. & L. Society* (Boston: Published by the O. O. and L. Society, 1906).

[88]*Ibid.*, 649.

[89]Donald Macfarlan, "A Reproving of Peruvian Bark," *Journal of the American Institute of Homeopathy* 40 (1947), 1-3.

[90]Donald Macfarlan, "A Reproving of Thuja," *Journal of the American Institute of Homeopathy* 55 (1962), 12-13.

[91]William Gutman, "Taraxacum Officinale — A New Proving," *Journal of the American Institute of Homeopathy* 49 (1956), 105.

[92]Anthony Shupis, "Cinchona Officinalis," *Journal of the American Institute of Homeopathy* 56 (1963), 395.

[93]Garth Boericke, "A Reproving of Cactus Grandiflorus with Laboratory Data," *Journal of the American Institute of Homeopathy* 39 (1946) 194-196, 212.

[94]Donald Macfarlan, "Reprovings of Medicines," *Journal of the American Institute of Homeopathy* 49 (1956), 135.

[95]Robert Koch, "Fortsetzung der Mittheilungen ueber ein Heilmittel gegen Tuberculose," *Deutsche Medizinische Wochenschrift* 17 (1891), 101-102.

[96]J. Kolmer, *Infection, Immunity, and Biologic Therapy*. Third Edition (Phila-

delphia: Saunders, 1923), 645. W. W. C. Topley and G. S. Wilson, *Principles of Bacteriology.* Second Edition (Baltimore: Wood, 1936), 910, 914. C. H. Dash and H. E. H. Jones, *Mechanisms in Drug Allergy* (Baltimore: Williams and Wilkins, 1972), 100.

[97]Dash and Jones, *op. cit.*, 14. P. F. D'Arcy and J. P. Griffin, *Iatrogenic Diseases* (Oxford: at the University Press, 1972), v.

[98]H. W. Crowe, *Handbook of the Vaccine Treatment of Chronic Rheumatic Diseases* (Oxford: at the University Press, 1931), 1-8.

[99]Walbum, "Metallsalztherapie. Sterilization des infizierten Organismus," *Zeitschrift fuer Tuberculose* 48 (1927), 193-216.

[100]A. King and C. Nicol, *Venereal Diseases.* Third Edition (Baltimore: Williams and Wilkins, 1975), 150.

[101]Crowe, *op. cit.*, 1-8.

[102]Zinsser, Enders, Fothergill, *op. cit.*, 478 (syphilis), 489 (tuberculosis).

[103]W. T. Vaughan, *Allergy and Applied Immunology.* Second Edition (St. Louis: Mosby, 1934), 361. Lawrence D. Dickey, *Clinical Ecology* (Springfield: Thomas, 1976), 544-553.

[104]*Science* 72 (1930), 526.

[105]*British Medical Journal,* 1943 (ii), 654.

[106]Fleming, *op. cit.*, 26.

[107]Zinsser, Enders, Fothergill, *op. cit.*, 344.

[108]Starling and Lovatt Evans, *op. cit.*, 1493-1494.

[109]W. E. Boyd, "Biochemical and Biological Evidence of the Activity of High Potencies," *British Homoeopathic Journal* 54 (1954). Reprinted in *Journal of the American Institute of Homeopathy* 62 (1969), 199-251.

[110]W. M. Persson, "The Principle of Catalysis in Biochemistry and Homoeopathy," *Journal of the American Institute of Homoeopathy* 23 (1930), 1055-1090.

[111]W. M. Persson, "Effects of Very Small Amounts of Medicaments and Chemicals on Urease, Diastase, and Trypsin," *Archives Internationales de Pharmacodynamie et de Therapie* 46 (1933), 249-267.

[112]*The Daily Telegraph,* August 19, 1954.

[113]M. Plazy, *Recherche Experimentale Moderne en Homeopathie* (Angouleme: Coquemard, 1967), 23.

[114]*Loc. cit.*

[115]*Ibid.*, 67.

[116]L. Kolisko, *Physiologischer und physikalischer Nachweis der Wirksamkeit kleinster Entitaeten, 1923-1959* (Stuttgart: Arbeitsgemeinschaft anthroposophischer Aerzte, 1959).

[117]Wilhelm Pelikan and Georg Unger, *Die Wirkungen potenzierter Substanzen* (Dornach: Philosophisch-Anthroposophischer Verlag am Goetheanum, 1965).

[118]Wilhelm Pelikan and Georg Unger, "The Activity of Potentized Substances. Experiments on Plant Growth and Statistical Evaluation," *British Homoeopathic Journal* 60 (1971), 233-266.

[119]Joseph Roy, "La Dilution Homoeopathique, sa Justification Experimentelle," *Le Bulletin Medical* 46 (1932), 528-531.

[120]Plazy, *op. cit.*, 19-22.

[121]*Ibid.*, 22.

[122]*Ibid.*, 68-72.

[123]*Ibid.*, 72.

[124]*Ibid.*, 73-78.

[125]Anna Koffler Wannamaker, "Effects of Sulphur Dynamizations on Onions," *Journal of the American Institute of Homeopathy* 59 (1966), 287-295.

[126]Anna Koffler Wannamaker, "Further Work with Boron Dilutions and Dynamizations," *Journal of the American Institute of Homeopathy* 61 (1968), 28-29.

[127]Hermann Junker, "Die Wirkung extremer Potenzverduennungen auf Organismen," *Pflueger's Archiv* 219 (1928), 647-672.

[128]J. Paterson and W. E. Boyd, "A Preliminary Test of the Alteration of the Schick Test by a Homoeopathic Potency," *British Homoeopathic Journal* 31 (1941), 301-309.

[129]N. P. Krawkow, "Ueber die Grenzen der Empfindlichkeit des lebenden Protoplasmus," *Zeitschrift fuer die gesammte Experimentelle Medezin* 34 (1923), 279-306.

[130]G. B. Stearns, "Experiments with Homoeopathic Potentised Substances Given to Drosophila Melanogaster with Hereditary Tumors," *The Homoeopathic Recorder* 40 (1925). Discussed in James Stephenson, "A Review of Investigations into the Action of Substances in Dilutions Greater Than $1 \times 10^{-24}$ (Microdilutions)," *Journal of the American Institute of Homeopathy* 58 (1955), 327-335.

[131]see note 85.

[132]Karl Koenig, "Ueber die Wirkung extremverduennter (homoeopathisierter) Metallsalzloesungen auf Entwicklung und Wachstum von Kaulquappen," *Zeitschrift fuer die gesammte experimentelle Medizin* 56 (1927), 581-593.

[133]Vladimir Vondracek, "Die Sterblichkeit der Kaulquappen in Ultraloesungen," *Zeitschrift fuer die gesammte Experimentelle Medizin* 66 (1929), 535-538.

[134]J. Jarricot, *L'Infinitesimal des Homoeopathes* (Lyon: Editions des Laboratoires P.H.R., 1951).

[135]*Journal of the American Institute of Homeopathy* 62 (1969), 230-231.

[136]Plazy, *op. cit.*, 25-40.

[137]*Ibid.*, 40-49.

[138]*Ibid.*, 51-62.

[139]*Ibid.*, 112 (L. Chedid, M. Parent, F. Boyer, and R. C. Skarnes, "Non-Specific Host Response in Tolerance to the Lethal Effect of Endotoxin" in M. Landy and W. Braun, eds., *Bacterial Endotoxins* [Rutgers, the State University, 1964]).

[140]*Ibid.*, 80-87

[141]*Ibid.*, 88.

[142]*Ibid.*, 88-95.

[143]O. A. Julian and J. Launay, "Psycho-Pathological Test on Animals by Reserpine and *Cicuta Virosa*, According to the Homoeopathic Laws of Analogy and Identity," *Cahiers de Biotherapie* (December, 1965). Reprinted in *Journal of the American Institute of Homeopathy* 59 (1966), 155-164.

[144]Plazy, *op. cit.*, 109-118.

[145]*Ibid.*, 62-67.

[146]I. A. Boyd, "Homoeopathy Through the Eyes of a Physiologist," *British Homoeopathic Journal* 57 (1968), 86.

[147]J. D. Van Mansvelt and F. Amons, "Inquiry into the Limits of Biological Effects of

110

Chemical Compounds in Tissue Culture, I: Low Dose Effects of Mercuric Chloride," *Zeitschrift der Naturforschung* 30 (1975), 643-649. Abstracted in *British Homoeopathic Journal* 64 (1976), 233-234.

[148]James Stephenson, "A Review of Investigations into the Action of Substances in Dilutions Greater than 1 x $10^{-24}$ (Microdilutions)," *Journal of the American Institute of Homeopathy* 48 (1955) 327-335.

[149]A. Gay, *Presence d'un Facteur Physique dans les Dilutions Homoeopathiques* (Lyon: Editions des Laboratoires P.H.R., 1951). A. Gay, *Etude Physique de la Dynamisation* (Lyon: Editions des Laboratoires P.H.R., 1952). A. Gay and J. Boiron, *Demonstration Physique de l'Existence Reelle du Remede Homoeopathique* (Lyon: Editions des Laboratoires P.H.R., 1953).

[150]Albert Brucato and James Stephenson, "Dielectric Strength Testing of Homoeopathic Dilutions of $HgCl_2$," *Journal of the American Institute of Homeopathy* 59 (1966), 281-286.

[151]Garth W. Boericke and Rudolph B. Smith, "Modern Aspects of Homeopathic Research" *Journal of the American Institute of Homeopathy* 56 (1963), 363-366; 58 (1965), 158-167. Rudolph B. Smith and Garth W. Boericke, "Modern Instrumentation for the Evaluation of Homeopathic Drug Structure," *ibid.*, 59 (1966), 263-280. Rudolph B. Smith and Garth W. Boericke, "Changes Caused by Succussion on N.M.R. Patterns and Bioassay of Bradykinin Triacetate (BKTA) Succussions and Dilutions," *ibid.*, 61 (1968), 197-212.

[152]Timothy M. Young, "Nuclear Magnetic Resonance Studies of Succussed Solutions," *Journal of the American Institute of Homeopathy* 68 (1975), 8-16. Timothy M. Young, "Anomalous Effects in Alcohol-Water Solutions," *Review of Iathematical Physics* 13 (1975), 10-12.

[153]James Stephenson, "On Possible Field Effects of the Solvent Phase of Succussed High Dilutions," *Journal of the American Institute of Homeopathy* 59 (1966), 259-262. See, also, G. P. Barnard and James Stephenson, "Microdose Paradox: A New Biophysical Concept," *ibid.* 60 (1967), 277-286, and G. P. Barnard and James Stephenson, "Fresh Evidence for a Biophysical Field," *ibid.* 62 (1969), 73-85.

[154]G. P. Barnard, "Microdose Paradox — A New Concept," *Journal of the American Institute of Homeopathy* 58 (1965), 205-212, at 211.

[155]See note 147.

[156]P. W. Bridgman, *The Physics of High Pressure* (London, 1949), 424 — cited in *Journal of the American Institute of Homeopathy* 59 (1966), 260.

[157]Timothy M. Young, "Nuclear Magnetic Resonance Studies" and "Anomalous Effects in Alcohol-Water Solutions."

[158]S. H. Kon, "Underestimation of Chronic Toxicities of Food Additives and Chemicals: the Bias of a Phantom Rule," *Medical Hypotheses* 4 (1978), 324-339.

[159]W. R. Houston, *The Art of Treatment* (New York: Macmillan, 1936), 22.

[160]*Chronic Disease, Advances in Diagnosis and Treatment* (June, 1974), 1.

[161]*Beitraege zur exper. Therapie* 11 (1906), H. 2, page 26. See, also, Brian Inglis, *The Case for Unorthodox Medicine* (New York: G. P. Putnam's Sons, 1964), 84.

[162]Hering, *Guiding Symptoms*, IV, 338.

[163]*New York Times*, May 27, 1974.

[164]Hering, *Guiding Symptoms*, IV, 334.

[165]*Ibid.*, V, 115.

[166]D'Arcy and Griffin, *op. cit.*, 48-50. R. I. Shader, *Psychiatric Complications of Medical Drugs* (New York: Raven Press, 1972), 25-47.

[167]Hering, *Guiding Symptoms*, III, 276.

[168]*New York Times*, July 28, 1972. *Washington Post*, May 12, 1976.

[169]J. H. Clarke, *A Dictionary of Practical Materia Medica*, I, 380.

[170]Hering, *Guiding Symptoms*, IV, 32.

[171]*Time*, December 11, 1964 (obituary of Sidney Haas, M.D., who introduced this use of *Belladonna* into allopathy). For the homoeopathic use of *Belladonna* in infantile colic see W. P. Baker, W. W. Young, and A. C. Neiswander, *Introduction to Homeotherapeutics* (Washington, D.C.: American Institute of Homoeopathy, 1974), 49.

[172]William Gutman, "Proving Symptoms of Rauwolfia Serpentina," *Journal of the American Institute of Homoeopathy* 50 (1957), 140.

[173]*Physicians' Desk Reference* (1975 Edition), 1454.

[174]Harris L. Coulter, *Homoeopathic Influences in Nineteenth-Century Allopathic Therapeutics* (Washington, D.C.: American Institute of Homoeopathy, 1973), 71.

[175]Jacques Forestier, "Rheumatoid Arthritis and its Treatment by Gold Salts," *Journal of Laboratory and Clinical Medicine* 20 (1935), 827-840.

[176]F. J. Wagenhauser, *Chronic Forms of Polyarthritis* (Bern: Hans Huber, 1976), 16. *Physicians' Desk Reference* (1970 Edition), 1177.

[177]J. H. Clarke, *A Dictionary of Practical Materia Medica*. Three Volumes (London: Homoeopathic Publishing Co., 1925), I, 223-234. Boericke, *Materia Medica with Repertory*, 96. Paul Talalay, ed., *Drugs in Our Society* (Baltimore: Johns Hopkins, 1964), 22.

[178]Hering, *Guiding Symptoms*, X, 433. John Henry Clarke, *The Prescriber* (Devon, England: Health Science Press, 1977), 231. *Physicians' Desk Reference* (1970 Edition), 1080. *Journal of the American Institute of Homeopathy* 46 (1953), 339-341, 343.

[179]Colman McCarthy, "A Minor Drug and a Major Problem," *Washington Post*, January 1, 1971.

[180]*Homoeopathic Recorder* 45 (1930), 184-186.

[181]Boericke, *Materia Medica with Repertory*, 14. H. C. Allen, *Materia Medica of the Nosodes* (Philadelphia: Boericke and Tafel, 1910), 4.

[182]*The Lancet*, 1965 (2), 104; 1968 (2), 426.

[183]Allen, *Materia Medica of the Nosodes*, 4.

[184]Clarke, *Dictionary of Materia Medica*, II, 420-421.

[185]Boericke, *Materia Medica with Repertory*, 427.

[186]A. M. Brooks, A. Agosti, *et al.*, "Inhibition of Gastric Acid Secretion in Man by Peptide Analogues of Cholecystokinin," *New England Journal of Medicine* 282 (March 5, 1970), 535-538.

[187]*Ibid.*, 565.

[188]Howard Haggard, *Devils, Drugs, and Doctors* (New York: Halcyon, 1929), 217.

[189]Clarke, *Dictionary of Materia Medica*, III, 1132.

[190]W. Gerlach, "Secale Cornutum gegen Gangraen," *Muenchener Medizinische Wochenschrift* 80 (1933), 1743-1745.

[191]Henry W. Eisfelder, "Some Homoeopathic Remedies in Modern Use," *Journal of the American Institute of Homeopathy* 49 (1956), 239-240.

[192]Harris L. Coulter, *Homoeopathic Influences in Nineteenth-Century Allopathic Therapeutics*, 60.

[193]Hering, *Guiding Symptoms*, IX, 248. H. A. Abramson *et al.*, "Production of Tolerance to Psychosis-Producing Doses of Lysergic Acid Diethylamide," *Science* 126 (November 15, 1957), 1020. C. Savage and L. Cholden, "Schizophrenia and the Model Psychoses," *Journal of Clinical and Experimental Psychopathology* 17 (1956), 405-413.

[194]Constantine Hering, *Wirkungen des Schlangengiftes, zum aerzlichen Gebrauche vergleichend zusammengestellt* (Allentown, Pennsylvania, 1837).

[195]Allen, *Encyclopedia of Pure Materia Medica*, III, 593. Boericke, *Materia Medica with Repertory*, 241.

[196]W. Buecherl and E. Buckley, *Venomous Animals and Their Venoms*, III, 458 and 466. Hering, *Guiding Symptoms*, IV, 487-488.

[197]Boericke, *Materia Medica with Repertory*, 454. Hering, *Guiding Symptoms*, VII, 530-531.

[198]*Science* 173 (30 July 1976), 387.

[199]Boericke, *Materia Medica with Repertory*, 453. Buecherl and Buckley, *op.cit.*, III, 450-451.

[200]Buecherl and Buckley, *op.cit.*, III, 456.

[201]Homoeopathic uses: viper venom as an anticoagulant in phlebitis (*Journal of the AIH* 56 [1963], 328), rattlesnake venom in thrombophlebitis (*British Homoeopathic Journal* LXIV, No. 1 [January, 1975], 36). Allopathic uses: prevention of Shwartzman's phenomenon and treatment of hemorrhage with 1 cc. of 1:3000 dilution of moccasin venom (*Ancistrodon piscovorus*) (*Journal of the American Medical Association* 104 [1935], 1066-1070), treatment of hemophilia with Russel's viper venom (*The Lancet* 1934 [ii], 985).

[202]Boericke, *Materia Medica with Repertory*, 63. B. F. Beck, *Bee-Venom Therapy* (New York and London: D. Appleton-Century Co., 1935).

[203]Boericke, *Materia Medica with Repertory*, 61. Buecherl and Buckley, *op.cit.*, III, 465-466.

[204]Boericke, *Materia Medica with Repertory*, 209. J. A. Pollia, "A Few Contributions to Modern Medicine that are Based on the Law of Similars," *Journal of the American Institute of Homeopathy* 44 (1951), 49-51.

[205]Paul Talalay, ed., *Drugs in Our Society*, 25.

[206]H. W. Eisfelder, "Clinical Homoeopathy," *Journal of the American Institute of Homeopathy* 45 (1952), 162-163. H. W. Eisfelder, "Today's Trend in Homoeopathy," *Journal of the American Institute of Homeopathy* 43 (1950), 221-222. M. Foxen, "Use of Streptomycin in Meniere's Disease," *Proc. Royal Soc. Med.* 47 (August, 1954), 671-672.

[207]A. Cier, J. Boiron *et al.*, "Experimental Diabetes Treated with Infinitesimal Doses of Alloxan," *Journal of the American Institute of Homeopathy* 62 (1969), 86-91.

[208]Susan M. Sieber and Richard H. Adamson, "Toxicity of Antineoplastic Agents in Man: Chromosomal Aberrations, Antifertility Effects, Congenital Malformations, and Carcinogenic Potential," *Advances in Cancer Research* 22 (1975), 57-155. In 1957 a case was reported of a woman with breast cancer which went into remission for nine months when treated with methylcholanthrene, a powerful carcinogen (*Journal of the American Institute of Homeopathy* 51 [1958], 15-16).

[209]Anselm L. Strauss, *Chronic Illness and the Quality of Life* (St. Louis: Mosby, 1975), 1.

[210]USDHEW PHS, *Limitation of Activity Due to Chronic Conditions. United States, 1969 and 1970* (Rockville, Md., 1973), 1, 3, 10.

[211]David Schottenfield, *Cancer Epidemiology and Prevention* (Springfield: Thomas, 1975), 4. *Time* (March 31, 1980).

[212]J. A. Del Regato and Harlan Spjut, *Ackerman and Del Regato's Cancer Diagnosis, Treatment and Prognosis,* Fifth Edition (St. Louis: Mosby, 1977), 2.

[213]*Journal of the American Institute of Homeopathy* 69 (March, 1976), 34.

[214]*Ibid.,* 45 (August, 1952), 171.

[215]*Ibid.,* 38 (May, 1945), 154-155.

[216]*Ibid.,* 45 (1952), 162-163.

[217]Louis Tuft, "The Skin as an Immunological Organ," *Journal of Immunology* 21 (1931), 85.

[218]Zinsser, Enders, Fothergill, *op. cit.,* 418.

[219]James Tyler Kent, *Lectures on Homoeopathic Philosophy* (Calcutta: Sett Dey and Co., 1961), 30. See, also, Herbert A. Roberts, *The Principles and Art of Cure by Homoeopathy* (London: Homoeopathic Publishing Co., 1936), 47.

[220]King and Nicol, *op. cit.,* 3.

[221]G. Vithoulkas, *The Science of Homeopathy* (New York: Grove, 1980), 111.

[222]Bastanier, "Koennen wir von der Homoeopathie lernen," *Deutsche Medizinische Wochenschrift* 55 (1929), 1041-1043. Coulter, *Homoeopathic Influences in Nineteenth-Century Allopathic Therapeutics,* 41-42. Editorial in *Minnesota Medicine* (August, 1971), 627.

[223]John Burry, "Topical Drug Addiction: Adverse Effects of Fluorinated Corticosteriod Creams and Ointments," *Medical Journal of Australia* (February 24, 1973), 393-396. See King and Nicol, *op. cit.,* 3 and 137, for discussion of the suppressive effects of antibiotics and mercurial medicines in syphilis.

[224]Alvan R. Feinstein, *Clinical Judgment* (Huntington, N.Y.: Krieger, 1967), 7.

[225]See the address by D. M. Martin, MD, to the American Academy of General Practice, as reported in *Time* (October 18, 1968).

[226]Paul Talalay, ed., *Drugs in Our Society,* 34.

[227]Pierce Gardner and Leighton E. Cluff, "The Epidemiology of Adverse Drug Reactions. A Review and Perspective," *Hopkins Medical Journal* 126 (February, 1970), 85.

[228]*Modern Treatment* 8:4 (November, 1971), 751.

[229]*Ibid.,* 944.

[230]*Chronic Bronchitis — A Symposium* (London: The Chest and Heart Association, 1959), 4.

[231]J. L. Achord, ed., *Chronic Inflammatory Bowel Disease,* 1.

[232]Quoted in *Journal of the International Academy of Preventive Medicine* 2: 2 (1975), 37.

[233]P. G. Quinton, "Analysis of 100 Consecutive Cases," *British Homoeopathic Journal* 35 (1945), 6-21.

[234]James Stephenson, "The Clinical Application of Homoeopathy — an Analysis of 100 Consecutive Case Histories," *Journal of the American Institute of Homeopathy* 49 (1956), 39-53.

[235]James Stephenson, "Twenty-Six Consecutive Pediatric Cases," *Journal of the*

114

American Institute of Homeopathy 54 (1961), 78-79. See, also, Edward M. Mead, "An Analysis of 31 Consecutive Homoeopathic Case Histories," ibid. 50 (1957) 271-273.

[236]E. W. Hubbard and James Stephenson, "Arthralgia — 100 Consecutive Cases," Journal of the American Institute of Homeopathy 50 (1957), 240-241.

[237]Raymond J. McGrath, "Vasomotor Rhinitis and Homoeopathic Treatment," Journal of the American Institute of Homeopathy 41 (1948), 211-213.

[238]James Stephenson, "Sinusitis — 33 Consecutive Cases," Journal of the American Institute of Homeopathy 52 (1959), 118, 120; James Stephenson, "Seventeen Consecutive Allergy Cases from One Month's Practice," Journal of the American Institute of Homeopathy 56 (1963), 326.

[239]Robert L. Redfield and James Stephenson, "Duodenal Ulcer — 35 Consecutive Cases," Journal of the American Institute of Homeopathy 51 (1958), 154.

[240]R. P. Patel, "Luffa Operculata in Asthma," Journal of the American Institute of Homeopathy 66 (1973), 219-222.

[241]E. W. Hubbard, "Headache — 51 Consecutive Cases," Journal of the American Institute of Homeopathy 51 (1958), 102; James Stephenson, "Headaches — 28 Consecutive Cases," Journal of the American Institute of Homeopathy 51 (1958), 130.

[242]E. W. Hubbard and James Stephenson, "Eczema, A Symposium of Collective Cases," Journal of the American Institute of Homeopathy 50 (1957), 206-211.

[243]T. Fergus Stewart, "Treatment of Coronary Disease in the Glasgow Homoeopathic Hospital," Journal of the American Institute of Homeopathy 59 (1966), 6-19.

[244]Paul Mossinger, "Treatment of Cysts with Silicea," Journal of the American Institute of Homeopathy 66 (1973), 225-226.

[245]R. G. Gibson, Sheila L. M. Gibson, A. D. MacNeill, and W. Watson Buchanan, "Homoeopathic Therapy in Rheumatoid Arthritis: Evaluation by Double-Blind Clinical Therapeutic Trial," British Journal of Clinical Pharmacology 9 (1980), 453-459, at 456-457.

[246]R. G. Gibson, S. L. M. Gibson, A. D. MacNeill, G. H. Gray, W. C. Dick, and W. W. Buchanan, "Salicylates and Homoeopathy in Rheumatoid Arthritis: Preliminary Observations," British Journal of Clinical Pharmacology 6 (1978), 391-395.

[247]"Report on Mustard Gas Experiments (Glasgow and London) by the Special Sub-Committee of the British Homoeopathic Society to the Ministry of Home Security (January 25, 1943), "Journal of the American Institute of Homeopathy 37 (1944), 47-50 and 88-92.

[248]W. J. Cross, "Veterinary Case Reports," Journal of the American Institute of Homeopathy 38 (1945), 215-217.

[249]M. Bardoulat, Precis d'Urologie (Toulouse, 1949).

[250]Plazy, op.cit., 119-121. The French have been particularly active in veterinary homeopathy: the September, 1979, issue of L'Homeopathie Française was devoted entirely to veterinary homoeopathy and contains 16 articles on such topics as: fever, mastitis, cough, diarrhoea, lithiasis, cystitis, dermatitis, joint troubles, rheumatism, paralysis, neuritis, and behavioral disorders.

[251]Ibid., 121.

[252]G. MacLeod, "Some Diseases of Farm Animals," British Homoeopathic Journal 61 (1972), 144-152.

[253]G. MacLeod, "Infertility in the Domestic Animals," British Homoeopathic Journal 64 (1975), 177-183.

254Anthony Campbell, "Homoeopathic Treatment of Ocular Infection in Guinea-Pigs," *British Homoeopathic Journal* 64 (1975), 68-69.

255Hans Brick, *The Nature of the Beast* (New York: Crown, 1962), cited in *Journal of the American Institute of Homeopathy* 58 (1965), 185.

256G. R. Henshaw, "Serum Remedy Diagnosis by Flocculation," *Annals of International Therapeutics* (June, 1969). See also, G. R. Henshaw, *A Scientific Approach to Homeopathy* (Hicksville, N.Y.: Exposition Press, 1980).

257Harris L. Coulter, *Divided Legacy: A History of the Schism in Medical Thought.* Volume III. Chapter VI: The Split in Homoeopathy — "Highs" vs. "Lows."

258L. S. Goodman and Alfred Gilman, *The Pharmacological Basis of Therapeutics.* Fifth Edition (New York: Macmillan, 1975), 351.

259*Ibid.*, 655.

260*Ibid.*, 728-730.

261F. J. Wagenhauser, *Chronic Forms of Polyarthritis*, 16.

262Paul Talalay, ed., *Drugs in Our Society*, 44.

263L. S. Goodman and Alfred Gilman, *The Pharmacological Basis of Therapeutics.* Third Edition (New York: Macmillan, 1965), 19

264F. W. Schueler, *Chemobiodynamics and Drug Design* (New York: McGraw-Hill, Blakiston 1960), 43.

265*Ibid.*, 71.

266A Bradford Hill, *Principles of Medical Statistics.* Ninth Edition (New York: Oxford University Press, 1971), 255.

267John N. Nodine and Peter E. Siegler, *Animal and Clinical Pharmacologic Techniques in Drug Evaluation* (Chicago: Yearbook Medical Publishers, 1964), 21.

268Roger J. Williams, "Normal Young Men," *Perspectives in Biology and Medicine* I (1957/1958), 97-104, at 98.

269Rinkel, *Specific and Non-Specific Factors in Psychopharmacology*, 137.

270Nodine and Siegler, *op.cit.*, 19.

271Ben F. Feingold, MD, *Introduction to Clinical Allergy* (Springfield: Thomas, 1973), 313.

# Addenda

# Addendum I
# Homoeopathic Dilutions Expressed as Powers of 10

| | | |
|---|---|---|
| $10^{-1}$ | 1X | |
| $10^{-2}$ | 2X | 1C (or 1CH) |
| $10^{-3}$ | 3X | |
| $10^{-4}$ | 4X | 2C (or 2 CH) |
| $10^{-5}$ | 5X | |
| $10^{-6}$ | 6X | 3C (or 3 CH) |
| $10^{-7}$ | 7X | |
| $10^{-8}$ | 8X | 4C (or 4 CH) |
| $10^{-9}$ | 9X | |
| $10^{-10}$ | 10X | 5C (or 5 CH) |

etc. to the Avogadro Limit of $6.12 \times 10^{23}$

Many homoeopathic remedies are used beyond the Avogadro Limit, i.e.

| | | |
|---|---|---|
| $10^{-24}$ | 24X | 12C (or 12 CH) |
| $10^{-400}$ | 400X | 200C (or 200 CH) |
| $10^{-2000}$ | 2000X | 1,000C or 1M |
| $10^{-20,000}$ | 20,000X | 10,000C or 10M |
| $10^{-200,000}$ | 200,000X | 100,000C or CM |
| $10^{-2,000,000}$ | 2,000,000X | 1,000,000C or MM |

# Addendum II
# What the Doctor Needs to Know in Order to Make a Successful Prescription

### James Tyler Kent, M.D.

*This article by Dr. Kent reviews the range of questions that homoeopaths may ask their patients in the case-taking process. No homoeopath will ask all these questions, but will ask those necessary to assess each patient's unique set of physical and psychological symptoms. Some of the terminology and concepts used in this article (written at the turn of the century) may today seem old-fashioned.*

We receive many letters from patients asking for medicine for some specified disease by name and not mentioning any symptoms upon which we can base an intelligent prescription. The homoeopathic physician has no remedy for the name of a disease. Homoeopathy is an exact science. It is based upon a natural law, and the true physician must prescribe in accordance with this law of nature. Homoeopathy has no specific for any disease by name, but it has a true specific for each individual case of disease. That is, homoeopathy does not treat fever, or any other disease, in the abstract, but applies medicine to the individual personality in that condition which produces or causes fever. To apply the homoeopathic remedy properly that condition of the individual patient must be known by the voice of nature speaking through symptoms. The beneficent Creator has ordained that every diseased condition shall be made known by certain symptoms, and whenever that same condition is present that same set of symptoms will also be present. Certain symptoms are always present in any given disease; these point alone to the name of the disease. In every given disease there is another class of symptoms peculiar to the individual and differing in some way from those of other cases of the same disease; these symptoms show the individual characteristics of the patient and point unerringly to the curative homoeopathic remedy. When these symptoms peculiar to the individual patient are known the homoeopathic remedy can be selected that will surely cure every curable disease, whether the disease be tumors, morbid growths, cancer or other skin diseases, or any form of chronic or acute disease peculiar to man, woman or child.

To accomplish this desirable result every case must be individualized, every symptom from head to feet, must be given, every variation from positive health must be known. Whatever is not as it should be is a symptom and must be recorded. This complete picture of the disease cannot always be given in a written communication, and hence, it is best for the physician to see the patient at least once. But as many patients wish to be treated by correspondence and, in fact, must be under certain circumstances, the same good result can be attained by the patient writing his most prominent, marked, peculiar and characteristic symptoms, especially those differing from other cases of the same disease.

To simply write "I have the headache", "the backache", "an eruption", or "a cough", would not be a guide in the selection of a homoeopathic remedy. Such statements are too general and do but little good. It would be mere guessing to select one of a possible hundred remedies to apply to the statements as above. But when you add to the general statement, "I have the headache," the individual peculiarities, "sharp shooting pains in the left side of the head and temple," you simplify the selection of a remedy very much. When you further add that the pains "always come on when the slightest cold air strikes the head," the pains are "much less when lying down and covering up the head warmly," and "much worse when rising up, walking about, or when the head becomes cool," you then state just what the physician needs to guide him. This is what is called "individualizing the case."

While taking the medicine it is necessary to abstain from every other kind of medicine, whether domestic, patent, or from another physician. Don't use camphor, perfumes, liniments, gargles and the like. Any of these may seriously interfere with the curative remedy. If worse at any time, and you feel that you must have relief, write the particulars to your own physician. Very often the curative remedy will cause an aggravation at first, or at the first menstrual period, but this is a good indication and should not be interfered with. Let the remedy have its perfect work.

The following suggestions and questions will aid the patient in giving such a description of his case as the homoeopathic physician must have to prescribe intelligently. These questions and suggestions should be read over till comprehended fully. Don't guess at the meaning; there is nothing here suggested, and no question asked, but that is most important. The success of the prescription depends largely upon your ability to describe your symptoms. ANSWER NO QUESTION BY "YES" OR "NO". Make your reply in full, giving all the particulars. Use your own language; the language used in these pages is merely suggestive. State your case simply, in full, with reference only to facts in the case. Do not refer to questions that do not refer to your case. No one case will have need to answer more than a small part of the questions propounded, but every patient must carefully read every line and word and reply to everything that has any bearing on the case in hand. Do not repeat the question in your letter, but merely state the fact in full. Pass by anything you do not comprehend. Consult the dictionary for any word you may not understand, so as to make sure of your statement.

The communications of patients will be held in the strictest privacy; no one will ever learn of your private troubles or symptoms through the agency of your physician. Therefore be perfectly free in your statements.

While taking medicine use common sense in diet. Avoid everything you know to be hurtful, or of which you have doubt. Avoid rich, greasy food, spices, cakes, pies, candies, tea, strong coffee, and food or drink after which you feel uncomfortable.

### Section 1. WHEN FIRST WRITING

Always state the name and address in full; give the age, occupation, married or single (how long married), the color of hair and eyes, the complexion, and any peculiarity of the patient as to form, appearance, size, etc., etc. Give your height and weight. State whether any near relative on father's or mother's side has died of, or been troubled with, consumption, asthma, cancer, tumors, scrofula, hives, erysipelas, skin diseases of any kind, or any other chronic complaint; also any peculiarity of the family on either side. Give a history of your own trouble—how it commenced and how long it has been troubling you, and any changes which may have taken place; what kinds of medicine you have used extensively; what you think caused the trouble; what name has been given to the disease; whether gaining or losing flesh or weight in the past few months; how often you have been vaccinated and the effect.

Always draw a line under the symptoms that are the most prominent and troublesome, or otherwise call attention to them so your physician may know them without doubt.

### Section 2. AFTER THE FIRST PRESCRIPTION

Always state when you began the last medicine; state any changes in the conditions or symptoms since taking the medicine, and the time of the change; mention the symptoms which are entirely gone, or are better, since taking the medicine, and all new ones. Specify the symptoms, and the old ones which return since treatment.

### Section 3. MENTAL SYMPTOMS

The symptoms of the Mind and Disposition are most important and should be carefully considered and reported. Give this section your particular thought.

How is your memory? For what is it poor? At what time is it poor? Do you remember what you read? Do you read with interest and pleasure? Can you apply your mind easily? In what way is your disposition changed during sickness? Are you mild, easy, gloomy, hopeless, obstinate, irritable, snappish, petulant, "real ugly" or sullen, cheerful, happy, or in what way is the disposition affected? Do you comprehend easily? Do you answer the questions of others promptly or slowly? Do you have anxiety, apprehension of the future, aversion to being looked at or touched, aversion to people, company or things; bashfulness, desire for company or solitude; desire for death; confusion of mind, delirium, discontent, disgust, dread of the future, of people, of animals or things; any peculiar feeling; mind full of crowding ideas, ill-humor, impatience, indecision, indifference, jealousy, too easily excited to tears or laughter, laziness, loquacity (inclined to much talking); disappointed love, melancholy, easy to be offended, feel like quarreling, sadness, scolding, screaming, sighing, taciturnity (silent mood), bad or persistent thoughts, or crowding of ideas, aversion to work, play, or anything else? How does the future look to you? Have you any delusions of any kind, or do you imagine you see things that have no existence, that your family has turned against you, that a man is under the bed or in the house, that someone is following or hounding you, that you are rich or poor, or will die in the poorhouse, hear voices, or that you are called, or anything else in this line?

Be very careful to give all these symptoms fully as they are very important. The questions and language here used are merely suggestive, being intended to lead you to give all your symptoms. The whole of this pamphlet is merely suggestive. It is not intended that the patient be restricted to the language or symptoms of the pamphlet. Give your case in your own language carefully and fully.

## Section 4. SENSATIONS

Sensations are also important and should be especially noticed.

For Sensations of pain, pain of all kinds, see Section 6. These special Sensations may occur in any part of the body, or internally, or in the head or extremities. Give the sensation in your own language to express it. No matter how simple, or even ludicrous, it is necessary to give it.

It may be like a mouse or bug crawling; like wind blowing into the ears or eyes; as if someone was pulling a hair; as of a blow on the back; as if the heart was grasped by an iron hand; as if claws were grasping the bowels; as of a splinter in the throat or flesh; like a string or thread on the tongue or in the throat; as if a joint were dislocated; as of a band or cord around the head; as though you had a cap on or hat; as of a plug in the ear or in some other place.

These are merely illustrations, a few that have occurred to other persons, and are given that you may understand what is meant by sensations. Always give the location as well as the sensation.

## Section 5. BETTER OR WORSE

This section refers to each disease, each sickness and to every symptom. No matter what the trouble may be it is necessary to refer to this section. Be sure that the aggravation or amelioration you notice is from the cause given.

The time of an aggravation or amelioration refers to the year, the month, the week, the day, the night, or the hour. State at what time your trouble, or any single symptom, is better or worse. State what season of the year, what time in the month, whether the phases of the moon cause either, what part of the week, what hour of the day or night the trouble or single symptom comes on, or is made better or worse.

Is there any position which you may assume that causes the trouble or any single symptom to be better or worse? It may be when you first lie down, or after lying down awhile, or on rising after sitting; standing, after standing awhile, or on sitting after standing; walking, walking much, walking in the house or in the open air, or in cold or warm air, or at night; running, running rapidly or slowly; when stooping over, after stooping, or on rising from stooping; leaning the head backward, forward, to one side, or leaning the head on the table or the hand; lying with the head high or low; lying in some particular position; crawling on the hands and knees; or some other of many possible positions.

Does anything cause the trouble or a single symptom to be better or worse? It may be reading, writing, music, ascending or descending the stairs or a hill, biting the teeth together, blowing the nose, before or after one of the meals, breathing, breathing deeply, when chewing food, when eating or drinking, closing or opening the eyes, looking up, down or sideways, from heat, cold, from warm or cold air, heat of the stove or sun, dry or moist air, going into the air or going into a warm room, sunlight or lamp-light, from excitement, fright, grief, sorrow, fasting, some kind of food or drink, motion or quiet, when nose is discharging or is dry, from gratification of the passions, scratching, rubbing, beginning of sleep, during or after sleep, loss of sleep, sneezing, before or during a storm, thunderstorm, snowstorm, swallowing food, drink or saliva, talking, singing, hearing others talk or sing, music, touch, turning over in bed, covering up or uncovering, wet, dry, windy, or cloudy weather.

The above is given to impress on the mind the great importance of noticing what may seem to be little things. Any one of these may be great or little, but your physician must be the judge of that.

### Section 6. PAIN

Give the exact location on the head, body, arms, hands, legs, feet, etc.; right side or left side; make this location as minute as you can.

State whether the pain remains in one place, or whether it

changes places; if moving or changing place state just how, and to what place it goes. Always mention the place where it starts and then where it goes, and how it goes. State how the pain makes you feel; the effect on you; how you act during the pain? Is there anything, any act, any position, any part of the day or night, application of cold or warm water, or dry heat or cold, any change in the weather, cold or warm air, or any other circumstance that causes the pain to be easier or worse, or removes it entirely? (See Section 5.) Is there any change in the appearance or feeling of the skin, flesh or bone after the pain leaves? What is your general feeling after the pain leaves? How does the pain come, quickly or slowly? Anything that seems to bring it on? How does the pain leave, quickly or slowly? What seems to cause it to leave?

What kind of pain is it? What does it seem like to your feeling or imagination? This is very important as there are various kinds of pain, such as cutting, boring, digging, bruised, sore, aching, biting, burning, cramp-like, dull, drawing, gnawing, jerking, labor-like, oppressive, paralytic, piercing, pinching, pressing, pricking, pulsative, stitching, shooting, tearing, violent, wandering (changing place), as from ulceration, as from excoriation or a raw place. Express the sensation of pain in your own language— just as it feels to you.

How much of the time do you have the pain? When is it likely to come on? When are you likely to be free from it? Is there any sore, eruption or swelling at the seat of the pain? Any change in the color of the place or in the usual appearance of the skin? Mention anything else about the pain that occurs to you, especially anything that appears to be unusual or singular.

### Section 7. DISCHARGES OF ALL KINDS

This refers to discharges from open sores, boils, fistulas, ulcers, etc., from the eyes, nose, ears, mouth, private parts, lungs, the skin, etc.

Give the quantity and the time or condition under which the quantity varies. (Section 5.)

Give the consistency, whether thin or thick, stringy, clotted like jelly, white of an egg, gruel, water, etc., etc.

The appearance, just what it looks like, the color, and the time or condition when the appearance varies.

The odor, what it reminds you of; whether the odor varies and the time and circumstances of the variation.

127

Whether it makes the parts sore, and in what way; whether the discharge has any effect on your feeling or strength; how long it has continued; whether the discharge comes and goes, and the time and circumstance of this variation. Whether it is sticky, forms a scab, etc. Mention anything else about it that you may notice.

## Section 8.  HEAD

Describe any pain as in Section 6. Describe any sores, lumps, or skin disease as in Sections 7 and 32. For sensation in head see Section 4.

Is the hair very dry or naturally moist? Does it split at the ends? Does it tangle easily,—how? Does it come out badly? Any dandruff? Quantity, shape and appearance. Is the hair oily or greasy? Does it break off, or mat together? Does it come out in spots or bunches. Be sure to give the exact location of any trouble of the head and whether internal or external.

**Dizziness.** Describe as in Section 5. What position, motion, or cause brings on the dizziness? What is the sensation? Do you feel like falling in any particular direction? Does it affect the sight? Do you feel as if swaying to and fro, in a circle, falling, rising, floating, as if bed were sinking, things about you were moving, etc. Give all the particulars.

## Section 9.  EARS

Describe pain as in Section 6. Describe discharges as in Section 7. Sores as in Section 32. Is the trouble inside, in the canal, or on the external ear? Right or left ear? Are you deaf? When and how can you hear best? When is your hearing poorest? How far from the right ear and the left ear can you hear a watch tick? Is your hearing getting better or worse? Can you hear better in a noise, on the cars, or riding? Is the hearing poor for the human voice or other noises or sounds? Have you too acute hearing? Do sounds hurt the ear or feel unpleasant? Have you any noises in the ear? Which ear? State minutely what the noise is like. Give any sensations in the ears as in Section 4. How does your own voice sound to you?

## Section 10.  EYES

Describe pain in the eyes as in Section 6. Discharges as in Section 7. Sensations as in Section 4.

Is the trouble in one eye or both? Which eye? Upper or lower lid? Inner or outer corner of the eye? Under the lid or on the outer side? Does one eye or both water? When? How much? Does the water make the eye or cheeks sore? How does reading or sewing affect the eyes? Are the eyes weak? Does the light of the sun or of a lamp hurt them or cause them to water? At what time are your eyes worse? Have you any peculiar feeling about the eyes? (See Section 4.) How long have you had the trouble? Have you or has any near relative ever had any trouble of the eyes? Have you ever used any eye-washes or salves? Can you refer the trouble to any cause? What appearance has lamp light to you? Has lamp light any peculiar circle around it? Are you near or far-sighted? Any swelling above or below the eyes? Any colored rings around the eyes? What color? Do you wear glasses? At what age did you begin to wear glasses? In case you do wear glasses, what would be the result if you did not? Have you had styes? On which lid and how many? Have you ever had a blow or other injury to the eyes?

## Section 11. NOSE

Is the trouble inside or outside, in forepart or back? For discharge, see Section 7. Do you blow out scabs or plugs? Give the size, colors, odors, consistency, and any other information about the scabs. Do the discharges make the nose or lip sore? Is the nose painful, swollen, or sore? (See Sections 6 and 32.) Do you catch cold easily? Do colds always affect the nose? Under what circumstances do you usually catch cold? For cold and catarrh report fully as in Sections 5 and 7.

## Section 12. MOUTH AND TONGUE

State whether the trouble is with the tongue or mouth, and what part of the mouth. Any sores? Give the location, appearance, color and size of the sores. Whether depressed or elevated? For the pain in the sores see Section 6. Is mouth or tongue dry or moist? Much or little saliva? Character, color, appearance and any peculiarities of the saliva? Thirst. (See Section 15.) Is the breath bad or foul? When does foul breath occur and what it is like? Any bad taste? When does it occur and what is it like? Any peculiar taste? Any peculiar sensation? See section 4. Is the tongue moist or dry? What is the coating on the tongue, its color and appearance? What part of the tongue is coated? Is there any peculiarity about the coating? How are the edges of the tongue? How is the tip? How is the back part? Does the tongue show the imprint of the teeth? Can you put it out of the mouth easily? When putting it out does it turn to one side or tremble? Any swelling or soreness under the tongue? Give direction and location of any fissures or cracks on tongue.

## Section 13. TEETH

Are the teeth sound or decayed? When did they begin to decay? Which teeth are decayed? What part of the teeth decay? What kind of fillings have you in the teeth? On what kind of plate are your false teeth? Are the front teeth smooth or rough on the edges like a saw? Are the teeth dirty-looking, yellow, black, or covered with mucus? Do they ache? (See Section 6.) Which teeth ache? What causes the teeth to ache? Cold air, warm or cold food or drink, when the body is cold or warm, when lying down, at night, etc., etc.? What relieves the aching? (See Section 5.) Is there any abscess at the root of a tooth? Do the teeth break off easily or crumble? Also consult Section 4.

Are the gums healthy? Do the gums bleed or recede from the teeth? Do you have gum boils? Are the teeth loose in the gums? Have you ever been salivated? Have the gums or teeth been in good condition since being salivated?

## Section 14. THROAT

Are you subject to throat troubles? Have you had quinsy, diphtheria, croup or sore throat? Have you had the throat burnt out, tonsils cut or lanced, or have you used strong gargles? Have you pain in the throat? (See Section 6.) Is there pain during swallowing solid food, drinks or saliva (empty swallowing)? Is the pain during swallowing or after? Have you pain when not swallowing? Have you any sensation or peculiar feeling about the throat? (Section 4.) Have you a desire to keep swallowing? At what time or from what cause do throat troubles come on? On which side of the throat is the trouble? Is it in the upper or lower part of the throat? Is there mucus causing hawking? When do you have to hawk the most? What causes the hawking? Do colds usually affect the throat? Is there any rattling in the throat? What is the appearance, color and condition of the throat? For swelling on the outer throat or neck see Section 32.

Is your voice clear? State wht may be wrong with the voice?

What is the effect of talking or singing on the voice? Is voice low, high or hoarse? Is the voice certain in speaking? Are you hoarse much of the time? Is the hoarseness painful? When does the hoarseness come on? What causes the hoarseness?

## Section 15. EATING AND DRINKING

Have you a craving for any special article of food? (Not merely a desire, but a feeling that you must have it.) Any aversion to any special article of food? Name the article in either case. Are you hungry much of the time or at any special time? Is the hunger or craving for food excessive? Have you no desire for food? Do you have hunger with aversion to eating? Do you eat without hunger? Does the food taste good? Has the food a natural taste? How do you feel before eating? Have you any bad effect from eating much or little? Do you desire little or much food at a time? Is there any special food that disagrees? Do you desire solid or liquid food? Do you crave you don't know what? Do you crave substantial food or dainties, candy, cakes, sweet things, sour things, etc., etc. Is the appetite even or variable? Does food satisfy you? Any trouble that always comes on after eating all you want, or after a little food? Do you eat hastily or slowly? Do you have sick stomach or vomiting after eating? Does eating aggravate other complaints? Are you sleepy after eating? Have you pain anywhere after eating? (See Section 6.) Do you suddenly lose your appetite or relish for food while eating, or at any time?

Are you very thirsty or thirstless? Do you wish to drink often or seldom? Do you want to drink much at a time, or little? What effect has drinking on you? Any trouble that always comes on after drinking? Do you crave any special drink? Do you wish hot or cold, or ice cold drinks? Do you feel badly after drinking? Does drinking satisfy you? Do you use tea or coffee? How much? Do you use alcoholic or other liquors? Do you use much milk? Does milk agree? Do you have sick stomach or vomiting after drinking? Does drinking aggravate other complaints? How does water, or other drinks, taste?

## Section 16. NAUSEA, VOMITING, ERUCTATIONS, ETC.

These terms stand for different things. It is necessary to make the distinction in writing your case.

**Eructations** (belching of wind). Is it frequent? When does it usually come on? Does it last long at a time? What relieves it? What makes it worse? Does it relieve the stomach, pain in any place, the throat, or do you feel better generally after belching? Have you pain anywhere before or during belching? Is the amount of wind great or small? Does it come up easily or with difficulty? Is there any other trouble that always accompanies it? Is there any bloating of the stomach or abdomen? Do you try to belch but cannot? Any nausea with it? Any taste with it? Acid, like almonds, like apples, bitter, greasy, fetid or foul, of food eaten, hot, rancid, salty, sweetish, etc.? State in your own language what the taste is like.

Have you gagging? When and under what circumstances? Any accompanying troubles? How does it affect you?

Have you at any time **heartburn** (an uneasy, burning feeling in the stomach?) Any accompanying troubles? How does it affect you?

Have you at any time **hiccoughing**? When does it come on? How often? Any pain? Any accompanying troubles? How does it affect you? What relieves it?

Have you at any time **regurgitation** of food (spitting up food in small quantity without vomiting?) Give particulars.

**Nausea** (qualmishness, squeamishness, loathing, sickness at the stomach). Where is the nausea located, or from where does it seem to come? Does it come and go, or is it constant when present? Does it always come on at a particular time? What seems to cause it? Is there any other trouble or pain that always comes before it or with it? How does it affect you? Describe the feeling in your own words. Does it come on suddenly or gradually? What relieves it? What makes it worse? Is there with it any faintness, fainting, dizziness, paleness, weakness? Do you vomit or retch with the nausea? Is there any sweating with it? Where is the sweat? Is the sweat warm or cold? Do you feel that it would relieve you to vomit? Is there simple nausea, or do you feel deathly sick?

**Retching** (to make an effort, or straining to vomit without vomiting). What causes it? When does it come on? Does it cause pain anywhere? How does it affect you? (Consult Nausea and Vomiting.)

**Vomiting** (emptying the stomach of its contents; puking). Give a minute description of what you vomit as to the appearance, consistency, color, taste, quantity etc.

132

Is it acid, acrid, like the white of an egg, bilious, bitter, black, bloody or blood, bluish, brown, clayey, like coffee grounds, cold, curdled, fecal, fetid or foul, fluid, frothy, glairy, greasy, green, jelly-like, milk, milky, mucous, musty, of pus or matter like rice water, salty, sweetish, watery, white, of worms, yellow?

Is it constant, copious, what you drink, what you eat, difficult, painful, periodic, spasmodic, violent, forcible, slow in coming on, sudden, coming on quickly?

When does it come? After eating, after drinking, after chill, from choking, from coffee, from cold, with colic, in convulsions, with cough, with cramps, during teething, with eructations, with eruptions on the skin, after exercise, during expectoration, in fever, from pain, from cold, when hawking, with heat, with hiccough, lying down, rising up, sitting up, standing, from motion, in the morning, when riding, after sleep, from smoking, before stool, on stopping, with sunstroke, swallowing, with thirst, with weakness?

Is there anything, any position, food or drink, or application that aggravate the vomiting, or relieves it?

Are there any accompanying troubles? How does it affect you? Make a full statement of anything else that may occur to you regarding the vomiting.

**Waterbrash** (pain or hot feeling in the stomach with a rising of water to the mouth). When does it come on? What is the amount? What is the taste? How does it affect you?

### Section 17.  THE STOMACH

The stomach is situated below the lower part of the breastbone, or beneath the depression known as the pit of the stomach.

In stomach troubles, indigestion, dyspepsia, etc., it is necessary to consult Sections 4, 6, 15, 16. For the part external to the stomach consult Section 32. For bloating consult Section 18.

### Section 18.  ABDOMEN

The abdomen is the belly, that part of the body between the chest and the pelvis.

In troubles of the abdomen consult Sections 4, 6, 15, 16. For the external abdomen consult Section 32.

Is there any bloating? When does the bloating come on? Is the bloating much or little, or tense, painful, etc.? Is the bloating over the whole abdomen or only in one place? What effect has it on you? Describe carefully any peculiar feeling in the abdomen as in Section 4. Is there any gurgling or rumbling? When does it come? How much of the time is the rumbling present? Is the abdomen depressed or full? Is there any soreness of, or oozing from the navel?

Describe rupture or hernia fully as in Sections 4, 5, 6, 32. How long has the rupture been present? How did it start? Is there any known cause of the rupture? Have you worn a truss or other appliance?

### Section 19.  URINE AND URINATION

The **bladder** is situated behind and extends a little above the bone in the middle lower abdomen. If painful describe as in Section 6. Describe any feeling or sensation as in Section 4. Have you ever had any blow or injury in this region? Have you ever retained the urine too long, or till it became painful? Any swelling or distension? Is it hot or inflamed? Any soreness or tenderness? Any bearing down pressure? Any sense of weakness? Any sense of uneasiness? Describe any trouble, pain or sensation in the urethra (the canal through which the urine passes). Describe any discharge from the urethra as in Section 7. Consult also the questions in Sections 36 and 37.

The **kidneys** are located on either side of the backbone (spinal column) in front of and more to the upper part of the small of the back, a little above the level of the navel. Describe any pain, sensation or trouble in the region of the kidneys as in Sections 6, 4 and 5.

**Urination** (the act of passing urine). Does the desire to pass urine come on at any particular time, or from any known cause? Is there any pain with the desire? (Section 6.) Does the urine flow easier in any particular position or under any special circumstances? Do you have desire to pass urine but cannot? Does it flow freely in a stream, or in drops? Does it flow at once or must you wait? Is there anything that you must do to help the flow start? Does it flow slowly or come in a gush? Is the desire urgent or can you easily wait? Have you involuntary urination during the day, at night, while coughing, sneezing, or at any time? What part of the night do you wet the bed? Is there any dribbling or leakage? At what time do you have most desire to urinate? Do you have to get up at night? How often? Can you pass urine without stool or stool without urine? Have you no desire to pass urine? Have you no passage of urine and yet no inconvenience? Do you feel the stream when passing? Does the flow intermit, start and stop? Any straining to pass? Is the stream even or divided?

Before urination. Describe any trouble, pain, etc., that always comes on just before the flow starts. Describe pain as in Section 6. Is there any burning before the flow starts? Describe and locate it. Is there any pressure? Any discharge other than urine? Be as explicit as you can as to these troubles.

During urination. Describe every trouble that accompanies the flow, or that comes on during the flow. Describe pain as in Section 6. Describe the burning minutely and locate it. Give the peculiar sensations as in Section 4. Do you have any chill, chilliness, any discharge other than the urine, faint feeling, pain anywhere, shuddering, etc.

After urination. The same as above.

**The urine.** Is the urine acrid (corroding), black, bloody, brown, burning, changeable in color, clear (limpid, no sediment or color), cloudy, like coffee, cold when passed, pellicle or cuticle or scum on it, dark, decomposes rapidly, decreased in quantity, flaky, foamy, frothy, like thin glue, dirty gray, greenish, high colored, hot, increased in quantity (profuse), jelly-like, light colored, suppressed, thick, turbid, violet color, watery, like whey, white yellow?

Mention any difference when first passed and after standing? What is the smell or odor? Do you pass gravel? Describe the sediment (the substance that falls to the bottom of the vessel) very carefully as to the amount, color, consistency, appearance, whether it varies, and other facts that you may notice. Does the sediment adhere tightly to the vessel? What is the color, consistency and appearance of that which adheres?

### Section 20. STOOL, DIARRHOEA, CONSTIPATION

**Stool** (whether diarrhoea, dysentery or constipation).

Character of stool: acrid, (excoriating), with air bubbles, balls, beaded, bilious, bloody, burning the parts, as if burnt, chalky, changeable, chopped, clayey, coffee grounds, copious, crumbling, curdled, diarrhoeic, difficult to expel, dry, dysenteric, fatty, fecal, fermented, fetid or foul, flaky, flat, fluid, foamy, forcibly expelled, frothy, glassy, like glue, granular, greasy, green scum, gritty, gushing out, hard, full of holes, hot, insufficient, involuntary, irregular, jelly-like, knotty, too large in size, lienteric (with undigested food), liquid, long, loose, lumpy, membranous, mixed, mucous, mushy, narrow in form, noisy (with wind), odorless, oily, painful, painless, pappy, pasty, like pea soup, periodic (at stated times other than each morning), pouring out, profuse, purulent (like matter), recedes (slips back), retained, retarded, like rice water, rough, like cooked sago, sandy, scaly, scanty (too little), like scrapings of intestines, sheep dung, shreddy, slender in size, slow, small in form, soap suds, soft, passes better when standing, passes better when leaning back, starchy, square, sticky, stringy, sudden in explosion, tar-like, tenacious, thin, thready, triangular, urging desire (cannot wait), watery, white, with worms.

Color of stool: ash colored, black, bluish, brown, changeable, dark, green, gray, liver colored, reddish, variegated, yellow, white.

When do you have stool? Afternoon, when coughing, after drinking, after eating, frequent, morning, on motion, from least movement, at night, at noon, before or during urination, after washing.

What trouble before stool? For pain see Section 6. For any other trouble locate and describe minutely. Chilliness, colic, faint feeling, fainting, flatulence (gas in bowels), passing wind, heat, piles come down, languor, lazy, nausea, sweat, tenesmus (pressing down in rectum), thirst, trembling, urging to stool (more than natural), vertigo (dizziness, vomiting).

What trouble during stool? For pain see Section 6. For any other trouble locate and describe minutely. Anxiety, bleeding, breathing affected, chill, chilliness, coldness, colic, disagreeable sensation, fainting, faintness, flatulence (gas in bowels), passing wind, heat, piles come down, hunger, nausea, nervousness, loss of fluid from privates, sleepy, straining at stool, sweat, bad taste, tenesmus (involuntary straining), thirst, urination, vertigo (dizziness), vomiting, weakness.

What trouble after stool? Same as during stool?

**Constipation.** See Stool in this Section. For pain anywhere describe as in Section 6. To what extent and when are you constipated? Are there any troubles that come on during or that accompany the constipation? Describe all troubles and locate. Do you feel better or worse during constipation? How often do you have a stool? Have you any desire for stool? How does the constipation affect the mind, the disposition, the head and the breathing? How long have you been costive? Has it followed any sickness, other trouble, or physic? Is it habitual or temporary? Does it always come on before or during any particular trouble, or any particular time? Is the child teething? Does it alternate with diarrhoea? Have you taken much physic or many pills? If so, state what kind. Have you used Hall's treatment of injections of hot water? Have you indigestion? Much wind in the bowels? The piles (see Section 21)? Liver or spleen trouble? A bad taste? Sore mouth? Nausea? Any skin disease (Section 32)? Vertigo or dizziness? Vomiting? What kind of appetite? What kind of thirst (Section 15)?

**Diarrhoea.** See Stool in this Section. Is it painful or painless? For pain Section 6. Consult Section 7. Most of the questions under Constipation (in this section) are suitable for diarrhoea.

What aggravates or ameliorates the diarrhoea? (Section 5) What seems to cause it? Acids, bathing, from cold, after drinking, during or after eating, exertion or work, riding, during sleep, after vaccination, after washing, any kind of weather?

Does it come on at any particular time of the year, month, day or night? Does it alternate with constipation? Is it chronic? Is the child teething? Does it weaken much? Do you lose flesh? Have you fever?

**Dysentery** (bloody flux). Same questions as under Stool and Diarrhoea. Describe more minutely the quantity of blood and mucus, and the character of the tenesmus (involuntary pressing down in bowels).

## Section 21. ANUS, RECTUM, PILES

**Anus.** Have you any trouble of the anus? Abscess, aching, beating, bleeding, boil, boring, bruised pain, burning, clawing, constriction, spasmodic contraction, cramping, crawling, cutting, darting, discharge (other than stool), dragging, drawing, dryness, eruptions, excoriated (chafed, raw), fissures (cracks), fistula (an opening beside the anus with constant discharge), dullness, heat, heaviness, inflamed (sore), injured, itching, jerking, pain (see Section 6), pinching, feeling as of a plug, pressure, pricking, prolapsed (protruding); state when and the effect, relaxed, sensitive, shooting, smarting (when?), soreness, sticking, stinging, stitches, straining, sweat, swelling, throbbing, tickling, tingling, ulcers, warts.

137

**Rectum.** (The intestine just within the anus.) Same questions as under Anus.

**Piles.** (Haemorrhoids). Describe the appearance of them. Color and shape. When do they come down? What causes them to come down? What relieves the pain in them? What aggravates them? How long have you had them? For the pain, see Section 6. For the discharge, see Section 7. Any peculiar feeling in them (Section 4)? Any bleeding? How much and when? Any pain or trouble anywhere else that accompanies the piles? Do they come with diarrhoea or constipation? Any itching, burning, smarting, soreness? Are they large or small? When and under what circumstances did you first have them? Have you ever had an operation for the piles? Have you ever had an injection of medicine into the piles?

## Section 22.  LUNGS AND BREATHING

Is the pain or other trouble in the chest muscles or deep in the lungs? For pain see Section 6. For cough and expectoration see Section 24. Do colds usually affect the lungs? Do you cough up anything? Do you have any difficulty in lying on either side or the back in lung troubles? Is there any rattling in the chest? Is there any consumption or lung disease in father's or mother's family? How many near relatives have died of lung troubles? Is there any soreness of the lungs? Any sensitiveness? Have lungs been injured by excessive exercise, running, etc.?

Do you have any trouble in breathing? By what is the breathing affected? In what position is the breathing affected? What position do you assume when breathing is affected? Do you have difficulty in breathing outward or inward (exhalation or inhalation)? Is breathing affected during or after sleep? While drinking?

For troubles of external chest see Section 32.

## Section 23.  HEART

Does the heart palpitate? At what time or under what circumstances does palpitation come on? Any trouble of heart after eating or sleeping? What kind of palpitation? Is heartbeat regular, loud, prolonged, purring, intermitting or skipping? Any other sound in the heart beside the beat? For pain in the heart see Section 6. Do heart and pulse beat together? How many beats per minute? Have you blueness of lips or fingers? Any difficulty in breathing in heart troubles? Any sensation in region of the heart? (Section 5.) Does motion or quiet affect the heart? Has heart ever been strained by excessive exercise, mountain climbing, etc.?

## Section 24. COUGH AND EXPECTORATION

What kind of cough have you? Constant, croupy, crowing, deep, dry, explosive, fatiguing, forcible, frequent, gagging, hacking, harassing, hard, harsh, hissing, hoarse, hollow, jerking, labored, loose, loud, moist, muffled, nervous, noisy, painful, in paroxysms (spells), periodic (at certain times), racking, rapid, rattling, ringing, rough, scraping, screeching, shaking, sharp, short, shrill, in single coughs, spasmodic, sudden suffocative, tearing, teasing, tickling (where?), tight, tormenting, violent, wheezing, whistling?

What causes the cough? Acids, anger, anxiety, coffee, from cold, crying, teething, while drinking, after drinking, as from dust, while eating, after eating, emotions, excitement, exertion or working, in fever, from fright, heart troubles, heat, indoors, out of doors, laughing, liver, troubles, least motion, mucus in throat or lungs, music, from nausea, odors, playing the piano, running, from smoke, stooping, talking, tickling (where?), dry weather, wet weather, windy weather, from yawning, going from open air into warm room, going from warm room into open air, when thinking of it, during study, sensation of sulphur fumes, feather, or what?

When does cough come on? Afternoon, evening, forenoon, lying down, sitting up, morning, night, noon, during sleep (does it waken you?), before arising in the morning, just after arising, before midnight, after midnight, early evening, and when going to bed, just after going to bed, in company, when alone, during the day, only at night, etc.?

Where does cough seem to come from? Abdomen, chest (lungs), back of mouth, windpipe, stomach, throat, etc.?

Where does it hurt you when you cough? How does it hurt you?

What effect has the cough on you? Must you hold your throat, chest, head, stomach, or any other part while coughing? For pain while coughing see Section 6.

Expectoration. Do you cough up anything? Describe it as in

139

Section 7. What does it taste like? Can you spit it out? Does it fly out of the mouth while coughing? Does it float in water or sink? Does it vary as to quantity, consistency, taste, etc.?

When do you expectorate and when not? Morning, noon, afternoon, evening, forepart of night, after part of night, at bed time, on arising in the morning, after arising in the morning? Under any other circumstance?

## Section 25. JOINTS

Locate the joint affected and the side the joint is on. For pain see Section 6. Describe any sensation or feeling as in Section 4. Any cracking on movement? Has it been out of place or dislocated? Has it ever been injured? Does it feel as if dislocated? Any eruption or sore about it? (Section 32). Is it inflamed, hot, swollen, sore, painful? Does it move easily? Is it stiff or is there no motion? Does the inability to move come from pain, or from what cause? Is it numb? Have you rheumatism now, or have you had it? Has it ever been sprained? Is it weak? Have you corns or bunions? Locate and describe as to pain and other particulars. Any trouble in walking?

## Section 26. MUSCLES

For pain in muscles see Section 6. For discharge from muscles (sores of any kind) see Section 7. Are muscles contracted, knotted, sore, stiff, any numbness, pricking, tickling? Report the sensations as in Section 4.

## Section 27. BONES

Describe pain in bones as in Section 6. Locate the bone affected. Has the place affected ever been injured, bruised or broken? Do your bones break easily? Is there any swelling of the bone? Describe the trouble carefully in all particulars.

## Section 28. BACK

For pain see Section 6. Also consult Sections 5 and 32. Especially describe the time or position in which the pain comes on. Also, what position or act (like pressure, lying on hard bed, etc.)

makes the pain better or worse. State carefully the part of back affected. Describe the sensations as in Section 4. Have you ever had the back injured in any way?

## Section 29. WOUNDS AND INJURIES

Have you had severe wounds or injuries in the past? Was your general health good after the injury? Have you had a hard fall? Describe it carefully. Is the wound a cut, tearing of the flesh, punctured, gunshot, sting of insect, a strain, or what? For discharge see Section 7. For pain see Section 6.

Give exact location. What caused the wound or injury? Did it bleed much, little or any? Did the wound heal readily? What is the appearance, color and shape of the scar? Does the scar give you any trouble? Does the scar change color at any time? What kind of insect stung you (if bad effect from insect sting)? What bruised the place? What is the color, appearance, extent of the bruise? What produced the burn (steam, hot water, fire, hot wax, etc.)? What is the extent and appearance of the burn? Is the burn deep or only on the skin? What produced the cut or laceration? Was either deep or shallow? Is the wound cold, or very hot?

## Section 30. BLEEDING

Give the cause of bleeding. Give the location or where the bleeding is from. Does the blood ooze, flow, or come in gushes? Is the blood thin or thick, clotted, lumpy, stringy, hot? Give color and appearance of the blood. Are you subject to bleeding? From what place? Have you ever been subject to bleeding? Does the bleeding weaken you? Are there any peculiar sensations or feeling that accompany the bleeding? Give all other known particulars.

## Section 31. MORBID GROWTHS, TUMORS, CANCERS, ETC.

In the treatment of these every symptom from head to feet must be known, therefore nearly every part of this pamphlet must be consulted and symptoms given as directed. These troubles can all be cured by the internal homoeopathic remedy when taken in time. To cut them out does not cure them. Cutting them out removes the effect of disease, but does not remove the disease itself.

141

It is like cutting off the tops of weeds—they will grow again, either at the same place or in another place. Months of careful treatment are required for their cure. When thus cured they will remain cured.

Give the exact location. Describe pain as in Section 6. Describe discharges as in Section 7. Describe the appearance, if on the outside. Describe the feeling to the hand, if on the inside. Give the size and general form. How long has it been coming? Is it hard, soft, yielding, movable? Any sensation in it? (Section 4.) Have you ever had any injury or blow on or near the place? Describe how it began and the growth. Has the growth been slow or rapid? Is it fast to the skin (if within)? Does it grow at any particular time or from any cause? What has it been called by other physicians? What treatment have you had for it? Ever had a surgical operation for this or any similar trouble? Have you applied any medicine to it locally? Has the treatment or local application made any change in it? Has any near relative on father's or mother's side had the same, or a similar trouble?

### Section 32. SKIN DISEASES

This includes all eruptions, pimples, sores, felons, abscesses, ulcers, carbuncles, boils, warts, morbid growths, tumors, cancer, and all kindred diseases, as these are all amenable to the homoeopathic internal treatment.

Consult Sections 4, 5, 6, 7, and 31.

Does the skin heal readily after an injury? Any roughness, chapping, sores from washing or cold weather? Are you subject to skin diseases, and for how long? Have any of your near relatives been troubled in the same way, or with any other skin trouble? Have you been vaccinated? How did it take, and what was the effect? Have you had the itch? What treatment was used for it? Have you had measles, scarlet fever, chicken pox, smallpox, mumps, or other similar diseases, and how did you get along during the sickness and afterwards? Have you ever had a surgical operation for the removal of tumors, morbid growth, etc.? (Section 31.) How do your nails differ from healthy nails? Have you hangnails? Ingrown toe nails? Have you foul, sweaty feet? (Section 7.)

How long has the skin trouble been present? How did it first start? Is the trouble sensitive to touch or pressure? Give the exact

142

location of places affected. Has the trouble been treated by local applications? Has any skin disease ever been suppressed or apparently cured by local applications? If so, what and when? What does the disease or sore look like? What is the appearance of the skin around the sore or under the sore? Is there any itching of the sore? What effect has scratching? Any scabs? What is the appearance and general form of the scabs? Any matter under scabs? (Section 7.) Describe any discharge from the sores as in Section 7. Describe pain as in Section 6. Any roughness of the skin? In what way is the skin different from healthy skin? Is there itching of the skin? (Section 5.) Give location, color and character of any spots or blotches on the skin, whether very small or large. Give location, color and appearance of moles or warts. What is the location, color, size, shape and appearance of any swelling? Any sensations on skin as itching, burning, pinching, crawling of insects or bugs, stinging or anything else? See Sections 4 and 5. Is the skin oily, shining, scaly? What is the color of the skin? Is the color permanent or natural? Describe pimples, little blisters, etc., as to location, size, contents, appearance, etc. Describe corns and bunions as to appearance, location and pain as in Section 6.

## Section 33. FEVER, CHILL AND SWEAT

Where have you flashes of heat? Have you flashes of heat and chill intermingled or alternating? Give location and time when either comes on. Is there shuddering? Are you inclined to be chilly generally, or in special parts? Where does the chilliness, or chill, begin and what course does it take? Do you like or desire the warmth or heat of the stove, sun or wraps? Do you feel better when warm or cold? Do you have thirst with the chill, fever or sweat? Do you have hunger with the chill, fever or sweat? At what time of day or night does the chill, fever or sweat come on? At what time is either the highest? At what time is either the lowest? What seems to cause the chill, fever or sweat? How long does the chill, fever or sweat continue? In intermittent fever (ague) do you have a distinct stage of chill, fever and sweat? How do you feel generally between the chill, fever and sweat, or after either? When having intermittent fever (ague) do you have hours or days when feeling perfectly well? Is one part hot while another part is cold? Do you have a chill as to any specified hour or day? Which predominates, or is worse, the chill, fever or sweat? Is the skin hot,

143

dry, moist, red, pale, cool or purple with the fever? Is there goose flesh with the chill or chilliness? What is the condition of the flesh during the sweat? What is the pulse rate? Is the pulse full, bounding, thready, skipping a beat, imperceptible, compressible?

Is sweat local or general over the body? Does any particular part or place sweat at any time. Do the covered or uncovered parts sweat? Is the sweat warm, cold, sticky, musty, clammy, foul, greasy, pungent smell, sour? What is the color? What color does it stain the clothing? Is sweat weakening? How do you feel during and after sweat? Do you sweat easily? Where, on what part do you sweat most?

Mention any other peculiarity of the chill, fever or sweat. Have you ever had ague? When, how long, and what medicine was taken for the ague? Have you been well since having the ague?

## Section 34. SLEEP AND DREAMS

State when and under what circumstances you are abnormally drowsy or sleepy. State when and under what circumstances you have yawning. Is the yawning painful or spasmodic? State all troubles or symptoms occurring before, during or after sleep, or when just falling to sleep? State all troubles that come on just as you waken and how you awaken; what awakens you during the night? Are you a sound, deep or a light sleeper? What causes the sleeplessness? When and under what circumstances are you sleepless? What seems to keep you awake when first going to bed, or when awakening during the night? Do you awaken often during the night? Is the sleep restful and refreshing? How do you feel when first awakening and on first arising in the morning? Do you take a nap or sleep during the day? Do you feel well after a sleep during the day? Are you easy or hard to awaken? Do you sleep quietly or toss and roll about during sleep? Do you like to sleep with the head high or low? Do you have the nightmare? Do you snore loudly? Do you moan, scream or make other noises during sleep? Have you sweat during sleep? Have you grating or grinding of the teeth during sleep?

Do you dream much? Do you remember your dreams? Do the dreams trouble you after waking? In what part of the night do you dream? Do you dream the same dream over the same night, or later? Are the dreams confused, pleasant, horrible, frightful, disgusting, disagreeable, vexatious, vivid? Do you dream of accidents, animals, cats, dogs, blood, business, church, death or corpses, dancing, danger, drinking, drowning, eating, falling, fire, flying, fruit, ghosts, horses, houses, being hungry, lightning, misfortunes, money, murder, of people, praying, being pursued, of quarrelling, riding, robberies, sexual pleasure, shooting, sickness, snakes, snow, talking, being thirsty, travelling, trees, urinating, vomiting, of water, weeping? Do you have day dreaming?

## Section 35. FOR WOMEN ONLY

In the treatment of diseases peculiar to women all symptoms from head to feet, and previous history, should be given. Local examinations and local treatment are seldom required and will only be made by the homoeopathic physician when really necessary. In these diseases, as in all others, nature speaks through symptoms which point to states and conditions well understood by the well-informed physician. These diseases, like diseases in other parts of the human economy, are amenable to the internal homoeopathic remedy; they should be treated like those hidden diseases where the eye of the doctor cannot penetrate, by the language of nature, by symptoms pointing to the pathological condition and the curative homoeopathic remedy. There is no need in the majority of cases for local applications, surgical operation, pessaries and supports, cauterization, removal of the womb or ovaries, and the accompanying shock to a true woman's modesty. All these diseases have been cured by the internal homoeopathic remedy, and they again may be by the intelligent physician. We are fully aware that there are conditions and states calling for surgical skill, but surgery should be the last resort. While it will require more time to effect a cure by medicinal means, it is certainly more pleasant, less repulsive to a modest woman, less dangerous, and more in accordance with the plans of a beneficent Creator.

It has often been said and demonstrated that homoeopathy is a woman's best friend. It respects her modesty, preserves her womanhood, relieves her of the many ailments peculiar to her sex and habits, and does it all more pleasantly. It might be parenthetically suggested that much of the suffering of woman arises from her habit of life and obedience to the demands of Dame Fashion.

In this section we allude only to those symptoms peculiar to women. No matter what the disease or trouble may be, the patient

145

should read all preceding sections and carefully give the totality of her symptoms as therein directed. Also, each part of this section should be carefully considered.

**Mammae** (the breasts). For pain see Section 6. For discharges see Section 7. For skin eruptions, spots, hard lumps, morbid growths, cancer, etc., consult Sections 31 and 32. Have you ever had abscess (beating) of the breasts? Have breasts ever been injured? Are breasts cold? Are breasts hard, swollen, inflamed, hot, sensitive, sore? Are breasts undeveloped (too small) or too large? Do breasts itch? Is there pain when nursing the child (Section 6)? Is there any fluid or milk in breasts other than when nursing?

Is there any trouble with the nipples or the part around them? Such as bleeding, burning, cracks, eruptions, gummy secretions, hard, inflamed, inverted or retracted, itching, pain (Section 6), redness, sensitiveness, soreness, swelling, ulcers?

**Genitals** (external sexual parts). Consult especially Sections 4, 6, 31 and 32.

Is there any trouble of the genitals? Biting, burning, congested, cracks, enlarged, eruptions, loss of hair, heat (feels hot), inflammation, irritation, itching, moisture, rawness, sensitiveness, smarting, soreness, stinging, stitching, sweat, swelling, tickling, tumors, ulcers, voluptuous sensation, warts. For any trouble, pain, etc., state all the facts as to aggravation and amelioration, Section 5.

**Vagina** (the canal which leads from the womb to the external orifice of the genitals). Especially consult Sections 4, 6, 7, 31.

State all the troubles of the vagina fully and particularly. Do not allow modesty to prevent a full statement. These matters are held in the strictest confidence.

There may be want of all feeling in the vagina, bearing down in the vagina, biting, burning, coldness, congestion, constriction and contraction of the walls, discharges (see Leucorrhoea), dragging, drawing, dryness, flatus or wind from the vagina, fullness, granulations, undue heat, heaviness, inflammation, irritation, itching, jerking, pain, pressing, pricking, prolapse or falling of the walls of the vagina, rawness, sensitiveness, smarting, soreness, stitches, swelling, ulcers, warts.

**Ovaries** (the ovarian region is to either side of the womb and above the groins). Especially consult Sections 4, 5, 6.

Always state on which side the trouble is. If an enlargement

146

or a tumor state pains minutely (Section 6), whether it increases or decreases, its relation to discharges from the vagina and menses, how long present, whether growth is rapid or slow, whether movable, and about the size. Have you ever been injured in the ovarian region? Did you have any trouble before marriage? Have others of your family, or your mother, had the same or similar trouble?

State all other trubles. There may be aching, bearing down, boring, burning, cramping, dragging, drawing, gnawing, grinding, heaviness, hardness, inflammation, itching (internal), jerking, numbness, pain, pinching, pressing, pushing sensation, sensitiveness, tenderness, shooting, soreness, stinging, stitches, swelling, throbbing or beating, twitching, twisting, etc.

**The Uterus** (the womb is situated in the middle lower abdomen, behind and extending a little above the bladder).

In this place it will be well to ask some very delicate, but important questions. A true answer to these may throw much needed light on the case. With these, as with all questions, no reply is to be made unless there should be something abnormal.

Were you led into the habit of masturbation (self-abuse) when a child, or later? To what extent did you practice it? Is there undue sexual desire? Is the sexual desire lost? Is sexual embrace painful or distasteful? Has sexual embrace been excessive? Are there any bad results following (within a few hours) sexual embrace? If married, how many children? If no children, do you do anything to prevent them? How do you prevent having children? It will be well to fully state everything abnormal about these things, and ask any questions that may give you needed light.

Especially consult Sections 4, 5, 6, 31, for womb troubles.

Do you have a consciousness of a womb? (Normally there is no feeling, hence no consciousness of any internal organ.) State the sensation if the womb seems not to be in the proper position. If there is pain or other trouble in any other part of the body which seems to be connected with the womb, state particulars and mention what relation there seems to be. Have you falling of the womb? If so, give the extent, the accompanying troubles, the time and cause, what relieves or aggravates (Section 5), and the effect upon you generally. To what extent have you worn a pessary or support, and what would be the effect if you did not wear any? For haemorrhage see Sections 7 and 30, and "Flow" under Menses in this Section. Have you ever received an injury in the region of the womb? Have you been ruptured or torn in childbirth?

147

In womb trouble there may be aching, bearing down (or a pushing as though everything would come out), burning, bursting feeling, contraction, congestion, cramps, cutting, discharge (see Vagina in this Section), distress, drawing, enlargement, fullness, heaviness, hardness, inflammation, labor-like pains, motion, neuralgia, pain, pressure, sensitiveness, soreness, spasms, squeezing sensation, swelling, throbbing, etc.

**Menses** (the monthly sickness or period). To insure a prompt cure it is necessary for patients to be very observing and report all symptoms as directed in other Sections. The interval between the the menstrual periods is 28 days, counting from the beginning of one period to the beginning of the next.

At what age did you have your first menses? Had you any trouble before or during the first period? Have you, at any time, had your menses stopped or deranged by getting wet feet, from a general wetting, from cold, fright, sickness, or from any cause? Have menses been irregular or painful since a particular time? Are your menses too frequent, too seldom, delayed, regular, early, late? How often do they come? For pain at the period describe as directed in Section 6, and Before, During, and After, in this Section. Do you have menses during the nursing of your child? Do you have the whites or nose bleed instead of the menses? How long do menses last? Does excitement or overexertion bring menses on? When does the flow increase, decrease, or cease? Afternoon, day only, evening, lying down, morning, motion, at night only, walking. Mention anything that affects the flow.

Character of the flow. Describe the flow very carefully. Acrid, black, bright red, brown, changeable, clotted or lumpy, copious, dark, excoriating (making parts sore), fetid or foul, greenish, gushing, hot (unduly so), intermitting as to flow, membranous (shreds), milky, mucous, odor (what is the odor?), pale, profuse, protracted (lasts too long), scanty, stringy, tenacious, thick, too thin, viscid, watery, dark clots in bright blood, etc. Give exact appearance and odor of the flow.

Before the Menses. It is very necessary to state whether the accompanying troubles of the menses are before, during or after the flow. We mention some of the more frequent troubles occurring at these times. Various troubles of the abdomen. Loss of or a very great appetite. Troubles of the back. Difficulty in breathing. Troubles of the chest. Chill. Chilliness. Costiveness. Convulsions. Cough. Delirium. Diarrhoea. Ear trouble. Eructations. Eruptions. Eye trouble. Face trouble. Fainting. Cold feet. Head troubles; headache. Leucorrhoea. Pains in arms or legs. Swelling, itching and soreness of the breasts. Mental changes (Section 3). Nausea or vomiting. Bleeding of nose. Ovarian troubles. Pain (Section 6). Restlessness. Sexual excitement. Urinary troubles. Great weakness or weariness. Describe all such troubles, and others, as directed in the various Sections.

During the Menses. This refers to the time from the starting to the ending of the flow. All the troubles mentioned as occurring "Before the Menses" may occur during the period, and many others. Describe everything as directed in other sections. Consult especially Sections 3, 4, 5, 6.

After the Menses. Many of the troubles referred to above may occur after the menses. Give all the complaints carefully as above.

**Leucorrhoea** (the whites). At what time does it come on? Is it all the time? Describe the color, consistency, odor and appearance of the discharge, and all accompanying complaints. Does it make the parts sore, raw or itch? What color does it stain the napkin or clothing? Notice what other complaints always come on or are worse when the leucorrhoea comes on or is worse. Does it corrode the clothing? Does it come on, or is it worse, before or after the menses? Are you excessively weak?

It may be acrid (corroding), albuminous (like white of an egg), biting, black, bloody, brown, burning, clear, cold, creamlike, dark, fetid or foul, like jelly, greenish, in gushes, honeycolored, lumpy, mild or bland, milky, mucous, opaque, profuse, purulent (mattery), ropy, scalding, scanty, smarting, causing soreness, starchy, sticky, stiffening the linen, suddenly coming and going, tenacious, thick, thin, thready, transparent, watery, white, yellow.

**Pregnancy** (during and after). There are many complaints incident to the pregnant state. These are all curable by the homoeopathic remedy, and when thus cured "labor" is always much easier because it is more natural. Treatment during this period is not only best for the mother, but is also best for the future health of the coming child, as well as for future pregnancies. The healthy woman will have no trouble and the minimum of pain in bearing children; normal labor is easy labor.

Report all these complaints as in the various sections of this pamphlet, but especially consult Sections 3, 4, 5, 6, 7. Nearly every abnormal condition of the pregnant woman will be found in the preceding sections.

Have you ever miscarried? How often, and what was the condition of your health afterward? At what month of pregnancy was the miscarriage? What caused the miscarriage?

For morning sickness consult Sections 15 and 16, and state how long pregnant.

How did you get along at your last confinement? Were instruments used? How long were you in labor? Was there any trouble with the after-birth or with the lochia (discharge)? How was your recovery from childbed? Describe any complaints you may have had following it.

Have you had milk leg? Do you nurse your child? If not, why not? Was the milk good and sufficient? How long after childbirth before having your menses? Describe any trouble you may have had during pregnancy or after childbirth.

**Climacteric** (the change of life). Describe any trouble which may arise during this period as directed in the various sections preceding, and especially consult Sections 3, 4, 5, 6, 7.

At what age did your mother or older sisters pass this period? If you are now passing it, at what age did it begin? Do you have flashes of heat? If profuse flooding, describe as directed in "Flow" in this section, and as in Section 30. If the past period, how long since? Did you have any trouble during the climacteric?

### Section 36. FOR MEN ONLY

For all complaints, whether local or general, the preceding sections should all be consulted and every symptom reported as herein directed.

For private diseases of men, homoeopathy offers a more radical cure than any other system of medicine. Local treatment by injections or applications is not curative, but suppressive. When so called local diseases are suppressed, or disappear under local treatment, they form the basis of chronic conditions which not only cause much annoyance and suffering, but are transmitted by heredity and may cause a lifetime of suffering to the children of lawful wedlock. Many persons have expiated the sins of the father by years of untold suffering. "Visiting the iniquities of the fathers

150

upon the children unto the third and fourth generation." The only sure and reasonable way is to eradicate the disease by internal constitutional medication. This is the real object of true homoeopathic treatment.

For all complaints, whether local or general, consult especially Sections 3, 4, 5, 6, 7, 32.

Answer the following questions, whether suited to your case, fully, and not by "yes" or "no," nor by a mere acknowledgement. Have you been addicted to the practice of masturbation (self-abuse) in the past? To what extent? Have you excessive sexual desire? Is sexual desire diminished or lost? Is there an aversion or repugnance to sexual embrace, or to women? Do thoughts of the sexual relation, or the desire for sexual gratification, crowd upon your mind? Does the presence of women cause sexual thoughts, or erections? Are your dreams persistently of sexual gratification, or of lewd women? Do you have sexual desire or teasing without erection? Are the erections incomplete or too soon lost? Has sexual embrace any bad effect on you mentally or physically? Is sexual embrace thrilling or has it no pleasure? Is sexual embrace complete or does the erection fail? Is the semen discharged too soon, or too late? Is the discharge of the semen painful? Do you have erections when riding in a carriage, or on the cars? Are you prompted to expose your private parts? Are you inclined to handle or manipulate your private parts? For pain in the parts locate and describe as in Section 6. Is there any unpleasant odor from the parts? Is there warm or cold sweat on the parts? Are there warts or growths on the parts? (Sections 31 and 32.) Do the parts feel natural and healthy, or do they feel weak? Is the penis shrunken, retracted, relaxed, lifeless, small, swollen, etc.? State the part of the penis affected as well as the trouble. Is the scrotum (bag) sweaty, contracted, itching, swollen, relaxed, or hanging loose, etc.? State any affection of the testicles (seeds). Describe any eruption or sores on the privates as in Section 32. Have you loss of semen (spermatorrhoea) at night, during stool, or at any time? What is the effect of this seminal loss? Is there a thrill with the seminal loss? Is the seminal loss during lewd dreams? Have you indulged your sexual appetite extensively? Have the parts been injured by a fall or a blow? Have you ever had a gonorrhoea (clap)? State the time and treatment, and the state of your health since. Have you ever had syphilis (pox)? State the time and treatment, and the condition of your health since. Have you had buboes, chancre, or ulcers? Have you had eruptions, sores, warts, etc., since having gonorrhoea or syphilis? Locate, state the character and the result. Have you gleet or any discharge from the penis? Describe as in Section 7.

A proper answer to the above, and a full statement of all troubles as directed in the various sections, are essential to the cure of any chronic disease wherever located. Do not treat this subject lightly, nor allow your modesty to prevent you telling the truth. All such information is held in the strictest confidence and is only asked for because it is of the greatest importance in the successful treatment of your case.

## Section 37. GENERALITIES

How are you affected by heat? How are you affected by cold? How are you affected by warm rooms? How much do you crave the open air? How restless are you? How are you affected by bathing? Feel better or worse by bathing? How does standing affect you? How does damp weather affect you? How do electrical storms affect you?

## Section 38. CONCLUSION

To mention all diseases, or all phases of disease, would make this pamphlet too long and confuse the patient. From what has been written the patient will see what is necessary to be given, and that all symptoms, whether great or small, are important. Nothing has been said of nervousness or weakness, though so common, but the patient will readily see that he is to give the cause of the nervousness or weakness, the condition, the time, the extent, what seems to relieve or aggravate and whether present all the time or only at stated times. So with every other condition or symptom.

This may seem to be useless to those who are accustomed to the practice of physicians who prefer to guess rather than to get at the bottom of the trouble. The old way may relieve the trouble for a little while; this complete and careful way is the only one by which diseases, especially chronic diseses, can be permanently cured. If the patient desires the surest way to a cure, to get full value for his money, he must himself go to some trouble to give his symptoms. The physician cannot be held responsible when important symptoms are withheld through carelessness or from design.

152

The reader will remember that all of this pamphlet refers to the sick, or the sick condition, and not to the well. Everything herein mentioned has been experienced by some sick person, even those parts that may seem very ludicrous. If these simpler symptoms were of no importance, why do some people experience them while others do not? The variations in sick conditions, even though slight, are most important to the homoeopathic physician.

For further information, write to your physician.

# Addendum III
# The Question of Clinical Trials in Homoeopathy and Allopathy

We commonly hear from allopathic physicians that if only the homoeopaths could demonstrate the therapeutic value of their remedies as "rigorously" as this is done in allopathy, specifically through "controlled clinical trials," many barriers to allopathic acceptance of homoeopathy would fall. In the following pages I want to scrutinize this idea from several different angles. Homoeopathy today is a rapidly growing system in all of the Western industrialized countries[1], and the problem of how to conduct clinical research is coming increasingly to the fore.

## I.

One source of confusion should be eliminated at the outset of any discussion on proving the efficacy of homoeopathy. The homoeopathic clinical trial differs radically from its allopathic counterpart in that it is not conducted for the same reason. The allopathic clinical trial is used to uncover new knowledge, for example, to determine whether Disease X is cured by Medicine Y, whereas homoeopaths derive such information solely according to the law of similars, that likes are cured by likes. This is a universal homoeopathic law applicable to all medicines and all diseased conditions. If the patients in a homoeopathic clinical trial do not improve, the appropriate conclusion would be either they were beyond recovery in the first place, that the correct homoeopathic medicine was not given, or that the level of prescribing during the trial was inferior. One could never conclude that Medicine Y was inapplicable to Disease X, since whenever the patient's symptoms resemble those of the proving of Medicine Y, it will be the indicated and effective remedy.

Clinical trials in allopathy are designed to disclose specifically whether Disease X is cured by Medicine Y. In homoeopathy new knowledge is developed primarily through the provings of medicines, not through clinical trials. The only reason for conducting clinical trials of homoeopathic substances is to demonstrate the efficacy of the homoeopathic system to allopathic observers. The outcome of any such allopathically based trial would be a matter of indifference to the homoeopathic community, since, as already noted, poor results would be ascribed not to the inefficacy of the medicine but to the prescribers' imperfect knowledge of homoeopathy, to the hopeless condition of the patients, or, as we will see, to the conditions of the trial which made it difficult or impossible to practice homoeopathy correctly.

If the purpose of such trials is to convince outsiders, then it is incumbent on the homoeopathic physicians involved in them to adhere as closely as possible to the familiar allopathic protocols while at the same time avoiding compromising the homoeopathic principles and procedures. Is it possible to reconcile homoeopathy and allopathy in this way?

This is a tricky question, since there is an ineluctable conflict between the homoeopathic and the allopathic therapeutic methods, sometimes concealed by superficial similarities. Allopathy assumes that "diseases" can be defined and classified and that the physician's task is to assign the given patient to his or her disease class. Homoeopathy, on the contrary, rejects the possibility of assigning the patient to such a class. Instead, it aims to *distinguish* the given patient from all others who may resemble him (or her) closely. Allopathy seeks the resemblance among patients, homoeopathy the differences. Hence they perceive quite different phenomena as significant for diagnosis and therapy. To summarize a lengthy analysis (whose details may be found elsewhere) allopaths view the physico-pathological and biochemical changes, together with their associated "common" symptoms, as fundamental and determining, while homoeopathy relegates all of these to a secondary position vis-a-vis the determining "peculiar" symptoms. *

This profound doctrinal divergence affects the attitudes of the two sides toward the organization of clinical trials. Allopathy, in theory, proceeds by assembling a group of patients suffering from some "disease," as defined by the common symptoms of the patients and their pathological and biochemical test results. The medicine or treatment undergoing trial is administered to all members of the group, while members of a "control group" of individuals also suffering from this disease receives a placebo or the preexisting mode of treatment. Success or failure is determined by comparing the outcomes in the two groups.

It is very important that the two groups be "homogeneous," meaning that all members meet the diagnostic requirements for the given "disease."

When allopaths seek to evaluate homoeopathy, they instinctively think in terms of assembling "homogeneous" groups of individuals suffering from the "same disease." To the homoeopath, however, this is entirely inapproriate: the allopathic test and control groups are not "homogeneous" at all, but thoroughly heterogeneous, since the "peculiar" symptoms of the group members will differ from one another, and it is these — not the "common" symptoms — which are significant for homoeopathic therapy.

In an allopathic clinical trial the pathological status of the patients is defined beforehand, and that diagnosis is assumed to be relevant during the whole course of therapy. The patient is assumed to have "Disease X" throughout the

---

*"The more common and undefined symptoms: loss of appetite, headache, debility, restless sleep, discomfort, and so forth, demand but little attention when of that vague and undefined character, if they cannot be more accurately described, as symptoms of such a common nature are observed in almost every disease . . . The most singular, most uncommon signs furnish the characteristic, distinctive and peculiar features . . . The more striking, singular, uncommon, and peculiar (characteristic) signs and symptoms of the case of disease are chiefly and most solely to be kept in view" (Samuel Hahnemann).

trial, and "Medicine Y" is prescribed for a sufficient period of time to demonstrate whether or not it is capable of curing "Disease X."

To the homoeopathic physician, however, such trial conditions would be considered inadequate. He could not legitimately treat a patient with the same medicine for an extended period of time—i.e., over the course of a lengthy clinical trial—if the patient's symptoms alter during that time, since changing symptoms usually require a change of remedy. It is this factor, in particular, that mitigates homoeopathic enthusiasm for the procedure known as "blinding" the physician—meaning that he does not know whether the given patient is receiving active medication or placebo. He cannot possibly evaluate the patient's progress without such knowledge.

Thus there are serious methodological difficulties involved in testing homoeopathic remedies according to allopathic standards. Nonetheless, these difficulties have been confronted with some success in two clinical trials conducted recently by R.G. Gibson and coworkers in Glasgow, Scotland.

In an initial trial, reported in 1978[2], a comparison was made among three groups of rheumatoid arthritis patients, one treated with salicylic acid, another treated with placebo, and a third treated on an individualized basis with homoeopathic remedies. The trial was single-blind: the patients did not know about the difference in treatment, while the physicians did. Furthermore, all members of the homoeopathic group were allowed to continue with their previous allopathic treatment if they so desired. Twenty-three out of fifty-four had discarded it within four months and thereafter were maintained on homoeopathic treatment alone, but thirteen others continued simultaneous allopathic treatment. This, of course, confused the picture, making it impossible to determine the precise contribution of homoeopathy.

In a subsequent rheumatoid arthritis trial, reported in 1980[3], two groups of patients were compared. The twenty-three patients in the first group received allopathic treatment plus a placebo, and in the second group twenty-three patients received allopathic treatment plus an individualized homoeopathic prescription (see pp. 88–89, above). The trial was double-blind, meaning that neither the physicians nor the

157

patients knew who was receiving the homoeopathic remedies during the course of treatment, blinding being ensured by keeping the prescriber in ignorance whether or not the given patient was in the test or control group. In other words, the prescriber could not know whether the patient for whom he was prescribing was actually receiving this medication or was, in fact, in the control group, i.e., receiving placebo. This meant, in particular, that "the doctors . . . did not know whether a failure of the patient to respond to their prescription was due to their inability to select the approriate remedy or to the fact that the patient was on placebo."[4]

Unfortunately, this trial was also marred by an insistence on having all patients, in both the test and control groups, continue allopathic treatment at the same time.

However, despite being hampered by having only partial knowledge of their patients and by the possible interference between ongoing allopathic therapy and the concurrent homoeopathic medication, Gibson and his colleagues were able to demonstrate the superiority of homoeopathy over an inert preparation in the treatment of rheumatoid arthritis. Thus, even though their trial design was imperfect from the strict homoeopathic point of view, they were able to achieve valid and significant results.

This trial protocol would seem suitable for future use, especially if modified to provide that the test group receive only homoeopathic remedies and the control group only allopathic treatment.

Thus, to answer the questions posed earlier, clinical trials of homoeopathic preparations can be performed following the allopathic protocol without doing excessive violence to homoeopathic principles and methods.

There is another group of trials mentioned by Scofield[5] which have compared a single homoeopathic remedy and a corresponding allopathic one in a given pathological state: *Rhus tox.* vs. Fenoprofen in osteoarthritis, *Arnica* vs. placebo in acute stroke illness, *Eupatorium perfoliatum* vs. acetylsalicylic acid in the common cold, *Arnica* vs. placebo in bruises, and *Staphysagria* vs. placebo in post-coital cystitis of women. The results were mixed, but, as Scofield observes, this procedure is, in any case, incorrect, as "a test of homoeopathy as a system, rather than a specific remedy, should be done" (p. 163). These kinds of trials violate the fundamental homoeopathic rule of individualization of treatment and are rather to be avoided than encouraged.

Since clinical trials comparing homoeopathy and allopathy will probably become increasingly popular, some thought should be given to modifying the protocols to bring them more into harmony with the spirit of homoeopathy. The controlled and double-blinded trial is not necessarily the only possible model. A.B. Hill, whose work in statistics made this trial possible, stated: "Given the right attitude of mind, there is more than one way in which we can study therapeutic efficacy. Any belief that the controlled trial is the only way would mean, not that the pendulum had swung too far, but that it had come right off its hook."[6] In particular, some more adequate substitute for "blinding" the homoeopathic physician should be developed; since he cannot prescribe accurately when he does not know if the patient's changed symptom picture is the result of his previous prescription or of some other factor. "Blinding," after all, is merely a technique for reducing—if possible, eliminating—observer bias. Any equivalent technique for reducing bias should thus be equally acceptable. The organizers of future trials should perhaps aim to develop bias-minimizing techniques which are more consonant with the spirit of homoeopathy.

## II.

The next question which may legitimately be asked is whether such trials are worthwhile. Some in our school feel that success in clinical trials will bring over large numbers of allopathic physicians to homoeopathy and that this will benefit the homoeopathic cause. But such an assumption may be wrong on several grounds.

The first objection to be made to such research is that, by discussing homoeopathy in allopathic language, we steadily erode and denature the essence of Hahnemannian thought and thus present homoeopathy in a somewhat false light. By encouraging physicians to concentrate on disease classes, such trials distract their attention from the individualizing concept which is integral to the homoeopathic doctrine. Practitioners attracted to homoeopathy by these kinds of research results could thus be ignorant of one of the central tenets of homoeopathy.

That this is not an entirely imaginary danger was demonstrated in the United States during the 1840's when homoeopathic success with the treatment of cholera enticed a large number of allopathic recruits who never clearly understood the Hahnemannian principles. They continued to practice allopathy using homoeopathic remedies and derided the efforts of Hering and Kent to preserve pure Hahnemannism. Ultimately they controlled the homoeopathic organizations and accepted a disastrous rapprochement, and, even, in some cases, fusion, with allopathy, leading to the collapse of American homoeopathy in the early twentieth century. There is danger that a major research effort might have an equivalent effect today, bringing into homoeopathy physicians who will diagnose the patient in allopathic categories and fall into such counterproductive allopathic habits as prescribing mixtures of remedies for presumed internal "causes," etc.

This danger is highlighted by Scofield's own comments. Although knowledgeable about homoeopathy, he betrays a certain ignorance on the subject of the individualization of treatment. He notes, for instance, that "the effectiveness of homoeopathic remedies may well be influenced by the sensitivity of the individual" (p. 180), that "only a minority of normal subjects are sensitive to remedies" (p. 217), that "homoeopathy would have us believe [that] this susceptibility to disease is a reflection of the disturbed equilibrium of the organism that is being treated" (loc. cit.), and "there is some evidence that not all organisms are sensitive to homoeopathic remedies. It is absolutely essential that this be clarified and, if found to be true, tests must be developed to identify those responsive to homoeopathic remedies" (p. 219).

These comments show that the author is in some confusion with respect to this central tenet of homoeopathic thought — so central, indeed, as to be a commonplace — that the sick individual is especially sensitive to the remedy which will act curatively in his or her case. The whole homoeopathic therapeutic method is designed to permit the physician to define the patient's sensitivity in the sense of selecting the remedy to which he or she will respond.

One can hardly understand what Scofield means when he calls for tests "to identify those responsive to homoeopathic remedies." If he means that some do not respond at all to any homoeopathic remedy, that would be news to the whole homoeopathic community. If he means identifying the remedy to which the individual uniquely responds, that is nothing more nor less than the practice of homoeopathy.

These preceding comments are designed merely to demonstrate how easily even persons with considerable knowledge of homoeopathy may be misled on important points of doctrine. This threat to homoeopathy's future should not be underestimated. It would be a pity if the success of a homoeopathic research program would have the same impact on the movement's future as the success of its practitioners combating cholera in the 1830's and 1840's.

Another reason for a cautious attitude toward this kind of research is that allopathic authorities have never extended recognition to the good work already done. Boyd's investigations in the 1940's which, as Scofield notes, many consider "a classic of homoeopathic research," (p. 178), although reported very briefly in the (British) *Pharmaceutical Journal*, never led to general acceptance of the homoeopathic microdilution. Are homoeopaths to keep repeating such research over and over again, at considerable expense, in the hope that some day the allopaths will deign to recognize it? Our resources might be better employed elsewhere.

Scofield observes that a fair number of the investigations described in his article were conducted at least as well as the average allopathic research project. And yet they could not be published in allopathic journals and of course have not elicited any allopathic response.

Here homoeopathy is confronted with a double standard. The allopathic physicians tell us, with some measure of condescension, that their professional self-respect prevents them from employing unverified procedures but that they would surely be receptive to homoeopathy once its techniques were verified by acceptable "scientific" (i.e., allopathic) protocols. And Scofield undertakes a heroic defense of this position, suggesting (pp. 217–218) "when this therapeutic system is opposed and disbelieved by the bulk of the scientific and medical establishment, the onus is upon the system to prove itself. It is, unfortunately, judged guilty until proven innocent . . . Homoeopathic research is a threat to conventional wisdom as it cannot be understood in conventional terms. Thus the smallest detail may become open to criticism in an effort to discredit the unexplainable. Greater caution is therefore required in the design and execution of [homoeopathic] experiments than in conventional science if the results are to gain any credence with the scientific community."

What Scofield fails to emphasize, however, is that investigations which are done impeccably (such as those of Boyd), and which cannot legitimately be criticized, are simply ignored in a general allopathic conspiracy of silence.

In fact, allopathic talk about willingness to look into homoeopathy as soon as it has been presented in acceptable protocols is for the most part mere puffery. Allopathic medicine, as an organized body, will *never* be able to accept homoeopathy, since the philosophical gap between allopathic Rationalism and homoeopathic Empiricism is too great. On this point homoeopaths should not be led down the garden path. Allopaths reject work done even in their own ranks when it is incompatible with the dominant Rationalist paradigm, the best example of this being the Arndt-Schulz Law. Although developed and expanded by allopathic physicians (Koetschau, Wilder, Hueppe), it is overwhelmingly ignored in allopathic pharmacologic texts. Rare indeed is the graduate pharmacologist who has even heard of the proposition that different dose levels of medicines yield qualitatively different physiologic effects. Why? Because this idea is incompatible with the mechanistic "law of mass action" which since the work of A.J. Clark in the 1930's has been the underlying assumption of allopathic pharmacology, even though its truth has never been demonstrated.

Of course, individual allopathic practitioners will espouse homoeopathy in the future as they have in the past. Every year a small group of allopaths goes through a transformation—which is more akin to a religious conversion than to a change of views based on the incremental accretion of knowledge. But these physicians change paradigms for a variety of different reasons and rarely out of conviction of homoeopathy's superiority based on the evidence from clinical trials. So there is at least some doubt of the value of such trials to homoeopathy's recruitment efforts.

## III.

Finally, our perspective on our own clincial trials will benefit from an awareness of the many difficulties encountered in allopathic clinical trials and of their rather poor quality.

A survey of the very extensive literature on these trials discloses a somber picture of virtually insurmountable practical obstacles to their correct conduct. Homoeopathic physicians who are aware of this literature will not be overimpressed by allopathic criticisms of supposed methodical errors in their own trial protocols.

Since this literature is vast, I will discuss the one requirement which, if unmet, deprives a trial of any value, i.e., the need for homogeneity among the patients in both the test and control groups.

After all, if the patients in the two groups are not all suffering from the "same disease," the trial has no point. And yet, to ensure that all are indeed sick with the "same disease" turns out to be quite difficult and probably impossible.

As already mentioned, homoeopathy maintains that each patient is different — hence, that group homogeneity is unachievable. The very idea of assembling several hundred patients with identical diseased states as determined by diagnostic and prognostic criteria is ridiculous. But this is the rock-bottom requirement for any allopathic clinical trial. If two modes of treatment, two medicines, are to be reliably compared, the patients must be identical in their diagnoses and their prognoses.

Thus, while allopathy in theory insists on the possibility, and necessity, of assembling homogeneous groups, experience since the inception of work on clinical trials in the post-World War II period demonstrates that this first step is the most difficult.

It has always been recognized that such investigations must allow for "some variation in each patient's unique biological and psychological makeup"[7], that the groups are homogeneous "except for the inherent variability of all biological material"[8], etc., but, at least initially, the authorities did not think that these idiosyncratic differences among patients would affect the outcome of trials. In 1966, however, after more than a decade of frustrating experience, A. Bradford Hill wrote that the unsatisfactory outcomes of many clinical trials was due to:

> biological variation of the human material with which we have to deal . . . Clearly our predecessors would not have got a very useful answer by applying one and the same treatment to a mixture of patients suffering from typhoid and typhus fevers before these two conditions were accurately differentiated from one another.[9]

Hill's pessimistic conclusion has been echoed by others.

> We were inclined to underestimate the extent of biological variation, which was such that a controlled trial was not always possible.[10]

> In discussions on the ethics of clinical trials there is usually a tacit assumption that the trial is scientifically sound. This is far from being the case in many instances, if only because clinical scientists often naively seem to believe that the material of the trial, which is human material, is reasonably homogeneous and that treated and untreated cases can be "matched," to use the jargon of modern clinical science. In actual fact it usually turns out to be impossible to control all the variables.[11]

Often lack of homogeneity is the result of failure to specify precise diagnostic criteria for inclusion of patients in the trial:

> Despite all the money put into academic institutions in the name of medical research, there has been very little careful categorization of patients. That information ought to have been obtained . . . Dr. Robert Gifford and I recently analyzed 32 reports of clinical trials where anticoagulents were used to treat myocardial infarction. Seventy-five percent of those papers contained no diagnostic criteria for what was meant by *myocardial infarction*.[12]

A 1983 review of 86 perinatal therapeutic studies concluded that only 34 (40%) provided "adequate subject description, while only 51% specified the "disease/health status of the subjects."[13] A 1984 review of 45 articles on antibiotic prophylaxis for abdominal wound infection found that six did not even define wound infection, while only 12 made a distinction between major and minor infections[14]. A 1984 survey of 16 studies of maternal-infant behavior as affected by contact immediately after birth found that less than half of the trials (47%) provided adequate "subject definition"[15].

The list of critical reviews of clinical trials, all observing that imprecision of criteria for the inclusion of patients has led to non-homogeneity of the test and control groups, could be prolonged indefinitely.

One reason for relaxing the criteria for entry into a clinical trial is that otherwise it is impossible to recruit a sufficient number of patients. Patient "accrual" into a trial is often a problem, and no one wants to exacerbate the difficulty of obtaining a sample large enough to support a statistically respectable conclusion.

The extreme difficulty of assembling homogeneous groups of sufficient size has been jokingly ascribed to the workings of "Lasagna's Law" — named after its discoverer, a well-known professor of pharmacology. This law specifies that "as soon as a trial begins, the supply of suitable patients becomes one tenth of what it was said to be before."[16] Or, in other words, "it is a world-wide experience that the supply of case-material is in inverse proportion to the facilities for studying it."[17] Lasagna himself has commented that "the problem of individual differences is indeed a challenging one, but it is no reason for paralytic despair."[18]

Whether or not a reason for "paralytic despair," this perennial problem of patient accrual has aroused the attention of pharmaceutical industry representatives — who are often more anxious to sell their drugs than to ensure strict adherence to clinical trial protocols. One of these commented on Lasagna's Law as follows:

> The most essential qualification of an investigator is that he should have, or have access to, an appropriate number of suitable patients . . . What causes the curious dis-

appearance of suitable patients as soon as we initiate a clinical trial? Usually *we* do. By "we" I mean medical advisors in the industry or anyone else who undertakes the detailed planning of a trial. In the interests of safety, ethical considerations, and accepted standards of safety, we stipulate patient selection criteria that exclude a high proportion of the available population . . . Everyone who writes about the design of clinical trials contributes to the operation of Lasagna's Law by insisting upon certain design criteria such as precision of diagnosis, homogeneity of groups, comparability of groups, and occasionally even matched pairs of patients . . .[18]

But even responsible physician-investigators admit the impossibility of perfect adherence to trial protocols:

Having been associated with numerous trials, we cannot recall any that have been entirely satisfactory. All have entailed some compromise short of the ideal. Perhaps the greatest difficulty in designing a trial is to decide the optimum conditions. If you wait until you can do it perfectly, you will probably never do it at all. We should not set our sights unrealistically high . . .[20]

The other side of the coin, however, is that relaxing the criteria contributes to non-homogeneity of the groups and vitiates the scientific value of the outcome. This is particularly true for mental illness:

Research into the nature of depression and its treatment by drugs is hobbled by the fact that *depressions* do not constitute a single homogeneous entity. Furthermore, interpretations of reported research data in this area have been confused by a general disregard for this heterogeneity and by a lack of precision and uniformity with respect to terminology.[21]

Where diagnosis is highly subjective and therefore imprecise, it is impossible to have homogeneous groups. Double-blind studies have been reported using antidepressants for treating depression. The matched groups contained endogenous depressives, schizophrenics who were depressed, and neurotic depressives. When heterogeneous groups are used, the therapeutic response is so variable that the responses of the treated and control groups depend too much on the random distribution of different classes of patients in them. No provision for this is made in the double-blind controlled design.[22]

Group comparability is, of course, not the only defective element in the design of allopathic clinical trials. Periodic evaluations by government agencies and professional bodies have discovered defective procedures, gross negligence, and even fraud and dishonesty in all areas.

In 1972 the U.S. Food and Drug Administration reviewed 155 clinical investigations and found that 74% failed to comply with one or more requirements of the laws and regulations, 50% failed to keep accurate records of the amount of drugs received from the sponsoring firm and distributed to test subjects, 28% failed to adhere to the test protocol, 23% failed to maintain records accurately reflecting the patient's condition before, during, and after the study, 22% did not retain case records as required, and 12% failed to supervise the study properly[23].

The following year, at the request of the General Accounting Office, the Food and Drug Administration inspected a sample of the work of 35 sponsor/investigators of new drug applications: "All 35 sponsor/investigators failed to comply with one or more of the FDA's regulations."[24] In its own 1976 report the General Accounting Office stated:

The Food and Drug Administration has neither adequately monitored new drug tests nor adequately enforced compliance with testing requirements. Consequently, it lacks assurance 1) that the thousands of human subjects used in such tests annually are protected from unnecessary hazards of new drugs, or 2) that the test data used in deciding whether to approve new drugs for marketing are accurate and reliable.[25]

Donald Frederickson, M.D., Director of the National Institutes of Health, observed in 1977 that of the 31,000 clinical trials conducted during the previous decade in the field of gastroenterology only 1% had been randomized; closer scrutiny of a sample of 100 led to the conclusion that *none* satisfied the requirements for a "convincing" trial[26].

The Kinslow Report issued by the FDA in the late 1960's when James Goddard was Commissioner, was a general assault on the drug industry for the poor quality of its clinical research and its failure to observe the requirements of the controlled trial.[27]

The Special Commission on Internal Pollution, an ad hoc committee with blue-ribbon membership, established in the United Kingdom in 1975, reported:

> Clinical trials of new compounds conducted by doctors are a shambles. Twenty percent of doctors doing such trials in the United States in 1973 whose work was spot-checked by the Food and Drug Administration were found guilty of a range of unethical practices, including wrong doses and falsifying records. Indeed, of all the reports submitted, the trial had not been carried out at all in about one third of them, in a third the established protocol had not been followed, and in only a third were the results of any scientific value.[28]

Louis Lasagna himself stated in 1971:

> The perfect trial has never been achieved. Most trials suffer from defects of one sort or another, such as the need to administer agents other than the one in question (because of ethically required fail-safe clauses), the breaking of the double-blind because of the production of side-effects by the active agent, differences in baseline variables in treatment groups in the study, and the occurrence of dropouts . . . The more practical-minded individual settles for a good deal less than the ideal, realizing that the latter is not attainable.[29]

One consequence of this has undoubtedly been the loosing of ineffective and harmful allopathic drugs on the market where they contribute to a rising tide of iatrogenic disease. Alvan Feinstein, professor at the Yale Medical School, has warned:

> Unless the scientific method of both innovative and conventional clinical therapy are made more sensible and re-

producible, the widespread distribution of modern therapeutic agents may provoke iatrogenic tragedies worse, individually and collectively, than any already known in medical history.[30]

In any case, the unexamined allopathic assumption that its medicines are subjected to rigorous scrutiny before acceptance cannot withstand rigorous scrutiny. Indeed, the Office of Technology Assessment of the United States Congress stated in 1978: "It has been estimated that only 10 to 20 percent of all procedures currently used in medical practice have been shown to be efficacious by controlled trial"[31].

Thus far homoeopathic remedies have demonstrated remarkable efficacy in clincal trials, despite being hobbled by the need to adhere to inappropriate allopathic protocols. At the same time, the allopaths themselves often seem unable to adhere to these very same protocols when testing their own medicines. If both sides are aware of these facts in the future, it will prevent a double standard from being applied — which can only benefit further clinical trials of homoeopathic remedies.

## Notes

[1]*Le Nouvel Observateur* (April 12–18, 1985) estimated that in France the homoeopathic volume of business is increasing at a rate of 20% per year.

[2]R.G. Gibson, Shiela L.M. Gibson, A.D. MacNeill, G.H. Gray, W. Carson Dick, and W. Watson Buchanan, "Salicylates and Homoeopathy in Rheumatoid Arthritis: Preliminary Observations." *Br. J. clin. Pharmacol.* (1978), 6, 391–395.

[3]R.G. Gibson, Shiela L.M. Gibson, A.D. MacNeill, and W. Watson Buchanan, "Homoeopathic Therapy in Rheumatoid Arthritis: Evaluation by Double-Blind Clinical Therapeutic Trial." *Br. J. clin. Pharmacol.* (1980), 9, 453–459.

[4]*Op. cit.*, 455.

[5]A.M. Scofield, "Experimental Research in Homoeopathy — A Critical Review," *British Homoeopathic Journal*, 73, 3–4, July and October, 1984. pp. 161–180; 211–226.

[6]Quoted in Joseph D. Cooper, ed., *The Philosophy of Evidence*. Washington, D.C.: Interdisciplinary Communication Associates, Inc., n.d. [1972], 11.

[7]A.D. Herrick and McKeen Cattell, *Clinical Testing of New Drugs*. New York: Revere Publishing Co., 195, 129.

[8]W.I.B. Beveridge, *The Art of Scientific Investigation*. New York: Vintage Books, 1957, 20, 28.

[9]A. Bradford Hill, "Reflections on the Controlled Trial," *Annals of the Rheumatic Diseases* 25 (1966), 108.

[10] *The Lancet*, 1964, ii, 949.

[11] *The Lancet* 1963, ii, 1156–1158.

[12] Joseph D. Cooper, ed., *The Philosophy of Evidence*, 59.

[13] Jon E. Tyson, Jaime A. Furzan, Joan S. Reisch, and Susan G. Mize, "An Evaluation of the Quality of Therapeutic Studies in Perinatal Medicine." *Obstetrics and Gynecology* 62 (1983), 100.

[14] Mary Evans and Alan V. Pollock, "Trials on Trial: A Review of Trials of Antibiotic Prophylaxis." *Archives of Surgery* 119 (1984), 110.

[15] Mary Ellen Thomson and Michael S. Kramer, "Methodologic Standards for Controlled Clinical Trials of Early Contact and Maternal-Infant Behavior." *Pediatrics* 73 (1984), 296.

[16] E.L. Harris and J.D. Fitzgerald, *The Principles and Practice of Clinical Trials.* Edinburgh and London: E. and S. Livingston, 1970, 43.

[17] T.B. Binns and W.J.H. Butterfield, "Clinical Trials: Some Constructive Suggestions." *The Lancet* 1964, i, 1150–1152.

[18] Paul Talalay, ed., *Drugs in Our Society.* Baltimore: Johns Hopkins, 1964, 93–94.

[19] Harris and Fitzgerald, *op. cit.*, 44–45.

[20] Binns and Butterfield, *op. cit.*, 1150.

[21] *Proceedings of the Institute on Drug Literature Evaluation: Philadelphia, Pennsylvania, March 11–15, 1968.* Washington, D.C.: American Society of Hospital Pharmacists, 1968, 74.

[22] A. Hoffer, "A Theoretical Examination of Double Blind Design." *Canadian Medical Association Journal* 97 (1967), 124.

[23] T.A. Vonder Haar and Mark Miller, "Warning: Your Prescription May be Dangerous to Your Health. *New York* (May 11, 1977), 53.

[24] *Ibid.*, 54.

[25] *Ibid.*, 54.

[26] "Proceedings of the National Conference on Clinical Trials Methodology, October 3–4, 1977, National Institute of Health, Bethesda, Maryland." *Clinical Pharmacology and Therapeutics* 25 (1979), 630–631.

[27] Joseph D. Cooper, ed., *Decision-Making on the Efficacy and Safety of Drugs*, Volume I. Washington, D.C.: Interdisciplinary Communication Associates, Inc., 1971, 83. Vonder Haar and Miller, *op. cit.*, 54.

[28] Special Commission on Internal Pollution, "Toward Assessing the Chemical Age." *Journal of the American Medical Association* 234 (1975), 509.

[29] Joseph D. Cooper, ed., *The Philosophy of Evidence*, 16.

[30] Alvan Feinstein, *Clinical Judgment.* Huntington, N.Y.: Robert E. Krieger, 1976, 40.

[31] U.S. Congress. Office of Technology Assessment, *Assessing the Safety and Efficacy of Medical Technologies.* Washington, D.C.: U.S.G.P.O., 1978, 7.